RICHARD O. DOLINAR, M.D. &
BETTY PAGE BRACKENRIDGE, M.S., R.D., C.D.E.

DIABETES

101:

Candy Apples, Log Cabins & You

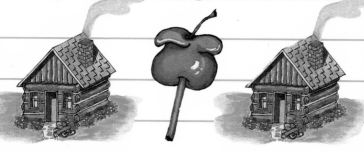

A Pure and Simple Guide for People Who Use Insulin

ISBN 0-937721-63-8

9 780937 721636

50795

RICHARD O. DOLINAR, M.D. &
BETTY PAGE BRACKENRIDGE, M.S., R.D., C.D.E.

DIABETES 101:

Candy Apples, Log Cabins & You

A Pure and Simple Guide for People Who Use Insulin

Library of Congress Cataloging-in-Publication Data

Dolinar, Richard O.
    Diabetes 101: A pure and simple guide for people who
use insulin.

    1. Diabetes--Popular works. (1. Diabetes.)
I. Brackenridge, Betty Page. II. Title
RC660.4.D65 1989   616.4'62   89-37754
ISBN 0-937721-63-8

Edited by: Donna Hoel
Design & Production: Wenda Johnson
Printed in the United States of America

10 9 8 7 6 5 4 3 2 1

Published by:

DCI Publishing
P.O. Box 739
Wayzata, MN 55391

Before You Begin

A tremendous volume of information is available to the person with diabetes. There are many books, mountains of pamphlets, myriad sheets and diet forms, rooms full of films, slides and tapes and a never-ending stream of committed health professionals gushing mind-numbing torrents of well-meaning words.

So why write another diabetes book? Great question. And we think we have a great answer. We wrote this little book because there is a need.

Not a need for another *War and Peace* of diabetes. A need, rather, for a brief and readable guide to important basic information used every day by people who take insulin to control their diabetes.

Some information about diabetes is vital to daily living. That information is in this book. And some additional liberating information about diabetes also is included.

But there is a good deal that is NOT in this book. There is so much helpful information about diabetes that it simply can't all be learned at once. Information that is very interesting but not needed for daily living with diabetes has not been included. And some information that is advanced and can only be mastered after a good deal of instruction and experience has also been omitted. There are many excellent sources for these kinds of information, and we encourage you to read them when you have the time. Today, though, read this little book.

We've been told it's helpful.

Betty Brackenridge
Rich Dolinar

Acknowledgements

Although this book carries the names of the two authors, in reality there are many others who have contributed greatly to its development. Our primary thanks must go to our patients who have taught us about the reality of living with diabetes every day and who have shown us the difference between what they needed to know and what we thought they should know.

Dr. Dolinar extends special thanks to the outstanding group of physicians present at Duke University Medical Center in the early 1980's who had a major impact on his interest in and approach to diabetes. They include Harold Lebovitz, MD, head of the Department of Endocrinology at that time; George Eisenbarth, MD, PhD, who provided many unique insights regarding Type I diabetes; George "Jay" Ellis, MD, who emphasized the importance of practical patient education and who modeled a dynamic problem-solving method of diabetes management; and Warner Burch, MD, who contributed his practical approach to patient care. Harry McPherson, MD, Frank Neelon, MD, Jerome Feldman, MD, Charles Johnson, MD, Mark Feinglos, MD, Marc Drezner, MD, and Titus Allen, MD, were very kind to share their many clinical "pearls of wisdom." And thanks also to Mrs. Johnnie Alexander who provided unique support in her own very special way.

And, finally, Ms. Brackenridge acknowledges an enormous debt of gratitude to the many colleagues who have contributed to this effort with advice or example; especially Keith Campbell, RPh, CDE, for technical consultation and friendly encouragement, Cathy Feste for faith, fun and her unique perspective, and Molly Miller for helpful editorial assistance when it was needed most.

SPECIAL NOTE: Consult with your doctor before making any changes in your diabetes care plan. The information contained in this book can help you become more active and informed regarding your diabetes management. But it is NOT a substitute for regular diabetes care by your physician or for in-depth diabetes education.

Table of Contents

Section I: The Basics

Section II: The Flashy Plays

Helpful Tables and Charts

SECTION I:

The Basics

Clowns to the left of me,
Jokers to the right.
Here I am, stuck in the middle with you.

Steelers' Wheel

CHAPTER 1

The Journey: Introduction

Not long ago, in a place not far from where you live, a young man named Mike began a journey. It seemed a simple enough quest. He was looking for a way to be healthy and live freely in his unique circumstances.

He seemed well equipped to find what he was looking for, but the goal still eluded him. He was bright, hard-driving and ambitious. He devoted long hours to the work he loved and was on the way up in his competitive field.

But the quest was necessary because, in spite of his many gifts, he had a problem: He had diabetes. And it was getting in the way of nearly everything he wanted and needed to do.

Having diabetes meant getting up early in the morning to allow time for an insulin injection, a blood sugar reading and a good breakfast. Mike couldn't get away with vaulting out of bed at the last minute, skipping breakfast and then sprinting for the train as his co-workers could.

Having diabetes meant his work day occasionally was interrupted by insulin reactions—periods of sweating and disorientation brought on by an unexpected drop in his blood sugar level. Once he even had one while making an important pitch to the top brass. He had to excuse himself to get something to eat. Now the young man worries that the boss may see him as weaker or less able than he once did.

Meals during the work day were a dilemma. Those business lunches eaten on the run didn't have much in common with the advice the dietitian gave him when his diabetes was diagnosed.

But they were a snap compared to dinner meetings with prolonged "happy hours." Discussing business over drinks could delay a meal for hours. How much should he drink? When should he take his insulin? What's more, the dinners were usually held in fine restaurants where the menus offered rich meals and extravagant desserts—not the best fare for a young man concerned with his health.

The list of challenges and frustrations seemed endless, but Mike was determined to find a way to take diabetes off the front burner. Surely his work and his social life would proceed more freely if that diabetes "pot" wasn't always at a full boil.

But Mike felt his doctor took a different view. At times the doctor would blame him for the frequent high blood sugars. The doctor implied, insinuated and at times even openly accused the young man of "cheating" on his meal plan. But sometimes the blood sugars were too high even when Mike had followed his meal plan to the letter. The doctor just wouldn't believe him.

At other times the doctor seemed to act as if it were Mike's **LIFE** that was getting in the way of his diabetes, rather than the other way around. And so the young man's quest began with a search for a new doctor.

His first attempt was with a doctor who seemed to solve all of his problems on the very first visit. With a slight smile and a wave of his hand he told the young man not to worry so much about tight control of his blood sugars.

"Just take this insulin dose, and I'll take care of everything else."

This seemed like the answer to the young man's prayers. It certainly was easier. What a relief not to be constantly worried about his blood sugar. But it wasn't long before he noticed his energy level was plummeting and his weight was dropping as well. He suspected his blood sugars were out of control.

One night as he was thinking about how hard it was to keep up his hectic schedule feeling the way he did, he ran across an article in a diabetes magazine. "A growing body of evidence strongly suggests that the long-term complications of diabetes may be prevented or delayed by excellent control of the blood glucose level," the article proclaimed. Mike knew it was time to resume his journey.

Next came a zealous physician who viewed normal blood sugars as the Holy Grail.

"Diabetes touches every part of your life, young man. Do exactly as I say and I'll have you in control in no time at all."

Then the doctor assumed control of every aspect of Mike's life. Each detail was put on a rigid schedule. Even occasional activities such as a game of tennis were to be entered on the schedule to allow for maximal control. The doctor's printed timetable was very different from Mike's usual schedule of work and sleep, but he was willing to try anything to get off the diabetes merry-go-round.

And so it seemed that every hour of the day was programed with some special activity related to his diabetes. As a result, Mike was forced to schedule fewer business appointments and even cancel meetings entirely on some days. Food was to be meticulously weighed and measured—an impossible task for someone who ate in restaurants nearly every day. But even more frustrating, the schedule for meals and snacks was at odds with his usual routine.

The young man's sanity was slipping away.

The last straw came when he returned to the doctor's office with the record book containing all of his painfully gathered finger-stick blood sugar readings. The doctor gave the book a cursory glance as he quickly thumbed through the pages, briefly looking at some and skipping others entirely.

Tossing the record book aside, the doctor gazed sternly at the young man. "These blood sugars aren't good enough yet. We need to tighten up your schedule."

Mike gasped in disbelief, but the doctor didn't notice. He was too busy adding more blood sugar readings to the schedule.

"You'll have to eliminate these tennis games too."

"But isn't exercise good for my diabetes?" protested the young man.

Without even acknowledging Mike's question, the doctor proceeded to "tighten the schedule," making even more extreme demands on the young man's time. When he finished, he turned abruptly and left.

Mike hadn't even had a chance to reply. He couldn't believe it!

Another appointment had ended, and he still didn't have answers to his many questions. He had taken a half day off work. He had fought traffic to get to the appointment on time. And then he had cooled his heels in a waiting room full of magazines so old they could have been unearthed in an archeological dig. But even after all this, he had had less than five minutes of the doctor's time and *none* of his attention. It was all too much. So was the bill.

It was time to leave . . . permanently.

Mike resumed his journey once again.

Many months, many doctors and many, many dollars later, he finally found the doctor he was looking for. The rest of this book is the story of what Mike then learned that put him where he belonged—in control of both his life and his diabetes.

WHEN YOU CONTROL DIABETES, IT WON'T CONTROL YOU!

I get by with a little help from my friends,
Gonna try with a little help from my friends.

The Beatles

CHAPTER 2

Riding the Bicycle: An Overview

One evening Mike's search took him to a diabetes lecture at a local hospital. He struck up a conversation with the woman seated next to him, and as they talked something became clear. Although she understood his problem, she did not have the same difficulties.

"Your doctors have been taking responsibility for controlling your diabetes," she said. "That doesn't work. What you need is someone to teach you how to take control for yourself. Try my doctor."

Since the woman seemed to be doing so well, Mike agreed to try just one more doctor. He called for an appointment.

A few days later, when they met for the first time, the young man blurted out his frustrations. "Doctor," he said, "I want to enjoy my life without thinking about diabetes every minute of the day. I want to work hard, entertain my clients and travel. I want to have my old energy level and stay healthy. I want to be myself again. Is that asking too much?"

"No, it's not. And if you're willing to work at it, I'm sure you can reach your goals."

"I'm glad to hear you say that, Doc. I was beginning to think I was in this all alone."

The doctor continued. "Do you remember when you were a child and learned to ride a bike? Managing your diabetes is a lot like that. It takes time. You didn't jump on a two-wheeler and pedal away the first time. In exactly the same way, it will take you a while to master the skills that will put you in control of your diabetes."

The doctor then pointed out, "No one else can ride a bike for you and no one else can control your diabetes. Ultimately, it's up to you. That's why it's so very important for you to master the skills yourself.

"Do you remember that great feeling when riding a bike got to be second nature? When you found you could ride it anywhere? So what if a cat ran in front of you or there were obstacles in your path? You made the necessary corrections and just kept rolling along. Eventually you probably even learned to do tricks on the bike. What a great feeling to ride with no hands, even though it gave your mom gray hairs!

"And the more you rode, the easier it became. Managing your diabetes will become much easier with practice, too. But first you need to learn the basics."

"What are the basics?" the young man wanted to know.

"Insulin, food, activity and timing. Once you understand these, you can play to win. You'll get feedback from blood glucose monitoring that will tell you how well your diabetes management efforts are working. Then you'll make corrections in the timing or amounts of insulin, food or exercise to produce even better control of your blood sugars.

"When you get that far, you're ready for the obstacles: delayed meals, eating in new places, getting sick and so on. You'll make the corrections you need and just keep rolling along."

"You mean I'll be able to do all of that myself?"

"Yes, and you'll even learn to do the diabetes equivalent of 'trick' riding. Like taking a European vacation or rafting down the Colorado River. When you've developed a bit more skill we'll talk about that.

"But your first job is to learn the basics."

LEARNING TO CONTROL YOUR DIABETES

- Takes Effort
- Takes Time
- Takes Practice

BUT...

It's Worth It!

Come on baby, light my fire.
                    Jim Morrison and The Doors

CHAPTER 3

Keeping the Fire Burning: Insulin

"Regulating your blood sugar is a lot like managing a fire in the fireplace of a log cabin out in the woods," explained the doctor. "Imagine that cabin is like a cell inside your body.

"Sugar in the blood is the fuel supply for your body's energy-producing fire, like the logs on the woodpile are the fuel for the fire in the fireplace. Insulin keeps the cabin door open so fuel can be taken from the woodpile and placed in the fireplace.

"Without insulin, the door closes and your body's energy-producing fire can't burn normally. That's why you must take your insulin every day, without fail. It's as basic to your survival as the food you eat, the water you drink and the air you breathe."

The doctor went on to explain that the exact amount of insulin a person with diabetes needs is determined by individual circumstances. The insulin dose needs to be tailored to fit those needs like a custom-made suit. Insulin requirements will vary— just as you sometimes need to tighten the belt or loosen the collar button, even when a suit is a good fit. And so the "fit" of the insulin dose has to be slightly adjusted from time to time by the person with diabetes.

Mike was unsure about the prospect of adjusting his own insulin. In the past, his doctors had always made all of his insulin adjustments.

"Don't worry," the doctor assured him. "We'll be doing this one step at a time. The minor adjustments to your basic insulin dose will be accomplished using a method I call "Dynamic Insulin Dosing[SM]." This is quite a change from the static dosing method used in the past. In static dosing, the doctor set an insulin dose for the patient, which remained unchanged for weeks or even months at a time."

Mike understood firsthand the drawbacks of static dosing. There had been times when his insulin dose had been set too high. Then he had experienced repeated low blood sugar reactions, with a progressive worsening of blood sugar control.

But at other times, the doctor had set the dose too low. Then he had gone for weeks with elevated blood sugars before seeing the doctor again for the needed insulin adjustment.

The doctor continued, "Now it's possible to accurately determine your blood sugars between office visits using meters designed for home use. This has revolutionized diabetes management and has made Dynamic Insulin Dosing not only possible, but very desirable."

"What is Dynamic Insulin Dosing, Doc?"

"It's a method you can use to adjust your own insulin between office visits. I'll estimate your dose based on all of the available information. But that dose will be a starting point, not an ending point.

"Using your blood sugar monitoring results and the Dynamic Insulin Dosing guidelines,* you'll be able to make stepwise adjustments in that insulin dose to improve blood sugar control gradually. Time won't be wasted waiting for your next visit with me. You'll be able to fine-tune the insulin to meet your needs as time goes along. You'll be in charge."

"That makes sense. But your approach is really different from the way my other doctors have done it," Mike commented.

"That's because we're now trying to mimic as closely as possible the blood sugar levels and control your body achieved on its own before you had diabetes. You've probably heard about research showing that good blood sugar control decreases your chances of developing the long-term complications of diabetes.

"No one type of insulin can work hard at all the times necessary to keep your blood sugar in that kind of excellent control. So to achieve near-normal blood sugars, we usually have to use more than one type of insulin and more than one shot each day. We'll be using both a short-acting (Regular) insulin, which will act in the first few hours after you take a shot, and a longer-acting (NPH or Lente) insulin that begins to work more slowly and stays in the blood-

*See page 21 for Dynamic Insulin Dosing Guidelines.

stream longer. The longer-acting insulins are made by adding protein or minerals to short-acting insulin so it is absorbed and used more slowly.

"With all of that going on, you can see it's really going to be important for you to understand when and how your particular insulins work. I'll always write your insulin doses so the units of Regular insulin come first. I want you to begin thinking of your doses that way too. That will remind you to always draw up the Regular insulin first when you prepare an injection. That's one way to make sure you don't accidentally get any of your longer-acting insulin into the Regular, changing its time of action."

"I guess I never really understood how or when to use my insulin. I would just take a shot, sometimes before breakfast, sometimes after. I didn't think it mattered."

"But injecting insulin is like shooting skeet," the doctor pointed out. "You have to 'lead' the target. That is, you have to shoot ahead of a moving clay pigeon in order to hit it. With insulin, you need to shoot (inject) ahead of the meal . . . for most people 45 to 60 minutes before the meal. This assures that insulin and food are available in the bloodstream at the same time."

"But I'll have a reaction if I inject that long before a meal. I've always been told to take my insulin when I eat. I've even taken it after meals at times, figuring that was a good way to avoid low blood sugar reactions."

"Strange as it sounds," the doctor replied, "NOT leading the meal with your insulin can actually increase your chances for a low blood sugar reaction."

The young man found that very hard to believe and said so.

"Let me show you what I mean," the doctor offered as he drew two graphs on a small piece of paper. Each graph showed curves representing the effects of insulin and food over time. The doctor pointed to the first graph and continued.

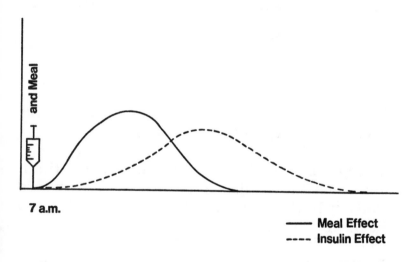

7 a.m.

―――― Meal Effect
- - - - Insulin Effect

"Not leading the meal with insulin is one way to produce 'curve mismatch.' This happens when the major action of your insulin occurs AFTER the major effect of food from your meal. Having a lot of insulin around when just a little food is available increases your risk for having a low blood sugar reaction.

"Now look at what happens when you lead the target:

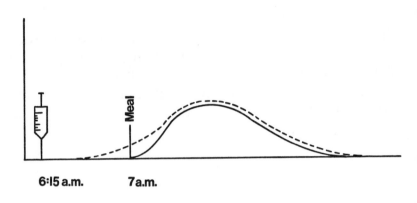

6:15 a.m.   7 a.m.

"Notice how the curves match more closely. This produces better blood sugar control."

"You may be right," the young man offered. "But it still seems if I waited that long to eat, I would probably have a reaction between the injection and the meal. It's happened to me before."

The doctor then explained that it takes quite a while for insulin injected under the skin to be absorbed and enter the bloodstream. There is a further delay between the time when insulin enters the blood-stream and the time the blood sugar level actually begins to fall.

"In short, Mike, when you had a reaction right after taking an insulin injection, it was being produced by the tail end of whatever insulin you had taken PREVIOUSLY, not by the most recent shot."

"Would it make a difference in all of this whether I was taking beef, pork or human insulin?"

"It wouldn't make any difference in what you should do. All the same theories apply regardless of the source of the insulin you're taking. But it might make a difference in the outcome—in how well we're able to control your blood sugar."

"Why would it make a difference in my blood sugar? I thought insulin was insulin."

"It makes a difference because your body recognizes beef or pork insulin as being different from human insulin. Even though the differences are very small, they can cause the body's immune system to make chemicals called antibodies to attack the animal-source insulin as a foreign substance. When that happens, the antibodies attach to the insulin and handicap its ability to do the job. In essence, the antibodies can 'tie up' some of the beef or pork insulin that's been injected so it's not available to lower blood sugar.

"The intensity of this effect in each person depends on the strength of the body's immune response to the animal-source insulin. The end result can be poor blood sugar control. So, since our goal is better diabetes control, today we're going to get you started on Dynamic Insulin Dosing using human insulin. I think you're going to see an improvement in your blood sugars because of these changes."

"OK, Doc, if you say so I'll give it a try." And off he went, determined to ride this bike called diabetes.

Insulin

1. Is needed every day: Missing a single dose could result in serious problems.

2. Is best taken at the same time each day.

3. Works best when taken 45 to 60 minutes before a meal.

4. With Dynamic Insulin Dosing and a doctor's assistance, can produce good blood sugar control.

DYNAMIC INSULIN DOSING ℠ GUIDELINES

Dynamic Insulin Dosing℠ is a method for making controlled step-wise adjustments in insulin doses to improve overall blood sugar control. It is used when there is no illness altering insulin requirements.

It is based on the following information:

Insulin Type	Injected	Has Major Effect	Effect Shown by Blood Sugar
Regular	before breakfast	between breakfast and lunch	before lunch
NPH or Lente	before breakfast	between lunch and supper	before supper
Regular	before supper	between supper and bedtime	before night snack
NPH or Lente	before or after supper	overnight	before breakfast

The following chart of insulin dose changes uses finger-stick blood sugar readings obtained at specific times during the day. It is based on a blood sugar "threshold" of 180 mg/dl. The threshold is the highest acceptable blood sugar value in the desired range of control a person with diabetes is trying to achieve. Your physician may adjust your threshold up or down depending on your specific needs. Your physician may also want to change the number of days you are to wait before making a dose adjustment, depending on the variability of your own blood sugar pattern and the level of control you have set as a goal.

Dynamic Insulin Dosing^{SM}

For **high blood sugars** not explained by illness or unusual diet or insulin. . .

If blood sugar is over 180 mg/dl for three days in a row:

BEFORE BREAKFAST
•*THEN*, beginning on day 4,
increase your evening NPH* insulin 1 unit.

BEFORE LUNCH
•*THEN*, beginning on day 4,
increase your morning regular insulin 1 unit.

BEFORE SUPPER
•*THEN*, beginning on day 4,
increase your morning NPH* insulin 2 units.

*or Lente insulin

BEFORE BEDTIME
•*THEN*, beginning on day 4,
increase your evening Regular insulin 1 unit.

For **low blood sugars** not explained
by unusual diet, exercise or insulin . . .

**If blood sugar is less than 70 mg/dl
or symptoms of a reaction occur:**

BETWEEN BEDTIME & BREAKFAST
•*REDUCE* tonight's NPH* insulin 2 units.

BETWEEN BREAKFAST & LUNCH
•*REDUCE* tomorrow morning's
Regular insulin 2 units.

BETWEEN LUNCH & SUPPER
•*REDUCE* tomorrow morning's
NPH* insulin 3 units.

BETWEEN SUPPER & BEDTIME
•*REDUCE* tomorrow evening's
Regular insulin 2 units.

---

*or Lente insulin

CHAPTER 4

Feeding the Flames: Nutrition

A few days later the young man returned to the doctor's office, but this time to see the diabetes educator. It was his first visit with her. She asked what part of his diabetes care plan he would like to learn more about.

"Eating," the young man exclaimed. "No doubt about it. Trying to figure out what to eat drives me crazy. So lately I've just been avoiding sugar and eating pretty much everything else I wanted. But I can see by my blood sugars that what I eat makes a big difference. Isn't there a simpler way than weighing and measuring everything I eat?"

"Well, as you've noticed, what you eat IS important to controlling your diabetes," the educator said. "But let's start with the basics: WHAT you eat, HOW MUCH you eat, and WHEN you eat it. Later, you may want to learn more about nutrition: how to read nutrition labels, what kinds of food can help cut your risk of heart disease, or how to make great tasting meals with less salt. Eventually learning and using a meal planning system like exchanges or carbohydrate gram counting may help you get even better blood sugar control. But for now, we need to focus on the big picture and start with the basics.

"WHAT to eat is actually pretty straightforward. A healthy diet is a healthy diet, whether or not a person has diabetes. You don't need special diet foods or way-out menus. The same foods that were enjoyable and 'good for you' before you developed diabetes are still your best choices. All of us—people who have diabetes and those who don't—will feel our best if we eat balanced meals including fruits, vegetables and grains with low-fat protein foods and dairy products."

"But I thought the most important thing about my diet now was to avoid sweets," Mike protested.

"It's true that eating large amounts of sugar and fat can contribute to poor control of your blood sugar and increase your risk of developing certain complications. But those weren't the best food choices BEFORE you developed diabetes either. And, by the way, they're still not great choices for people who DON'T have diabetes."

The educator pointed out that avoiding or limiting foods that have a high content of fat (such as fried foods, gravies, butter and salad dressing) and sugar (such as pies, candies, frostings and regular soda pop) is a good first step toward a healthier diet. Food labels often provide the information needed to help you avoid these ingredients.

"Besides taking it easy on fats and sugars, keep in mind that it's best if each meal and snack is composed of a variety of foods. Combinations that provide carbohydrate, protein and small amounts of fat will produce more stable blood sugar patterns."

She then handed Mike a sheet of paper that read:

INCLUDE FOODS FROM BOTH GROUPS IN MEALS AND SNACKS

CARBOHYDRATE	PROTEIN
Bread	Meat
Cereal	Milk*
Potatoes	Fish
Rice	Chicken
Beans*	Cheese
Crackers	Beans*
Fruit	Tofu
Milk*	Eggs

*Milk and beans contain both carbohydrate and protein.

"As to HOW MUCH to eat, there are two things to consider: first, the total amount of food you eat, and second, the amount you eat at any one time.

"First, let's talk about the total amount of food you need each day. The right calorie level for you is determined by your size, your level of physical activity, and whether you're a man or a woman, NOT by the fact that you have diabetes or how much insulin you're taking.

"You should be eating enough to maintain your normal weight and provide enough energy for your level of activity. A common mistake is to try to bring down a high blood sugar reading by delaying, reducing or even skipping meals or snacks. This is not the best way to manage your food intake. It may lead to a low blood sugar reaction later if insulin is available but there are no 'logs on the woodpile.' In Type I diabetes—the kind you have—you can't get good day-to-day control by eating less than you really need."

"You mean I have a different kind of diabetes than other people?"

"Yes. But I think it helps to think of diabetes not as something you HAVE but as something you DON'T have. Everyone with diabetes has lost the ability to automatically regulate his or her blood sugar level. What the body used to do automatically now needs to be done manually, no matter what type of diabetes you have.

"And there are several different types. But Type I and Type II are the most common. In the past, Type I diabetes was called *juvenile diabetes* and Type II diabetes was referred to as *adult-onset.*"
"What's the difference?"

"In Type I diabetes, cells that make insulin have been destroyed. We believe this happens because of a problem with the immune system. The immune system normally defends us against infection, but in some people it seems to backfire and destroy the cells in the pancreas, the organ that makes insulin. We don't know why this happens, but the result is that these people become unable to make enough insulin. Then they need to take injected insulin.

"Type II diabetes is a different disease. Many people with Type II diabetes make as much insulin as people who don't have diabetes. Sometimes they make more! The problem is that the insulin is not used effectively. Remember how we explained that insulin keeps the door to the log cabin open, allowing fuel to be brought in to the fire? You can think of the person with Type II diabetes as having very rusty hinges on the door, making it hard to open. This type of diabetes often can be treated effectively with diet, weight reduction and pills, since all of these help in some way to 'oil' the rusty hinges, so the door works better."

"Do people with Type II diabetes ever need to take insulin?"

"Some do and some don't. Generally we try first to get good blood sugar control using a weight reduction diet. If nutrition alone doesn't produce blood sugar control, a pill that helps the body make and use its own insulin better may be added. But if the blood sugars are still above normal with a good diet plan and pills, we often go ahead and add insulin as well."

"How can you tell the difference between the types of diabetes?"

"Usually people with Type I diabetes have had at least one episode of a condition called diabetic ketoacidosis. Those with Type II usually have not experienced that."

"What's diabetic ketoacidosis?"

"Let's hold off on that for a little while, Mike. Right now let's get back to your original questions about food. We had been talking about how MUCH food you need each day. Now let's spend a little time on how much you should eat at one time.

"Think again about the example of building a fire in your log cabin. If you were depending on that fire to keep you warm throughout a freezing winter night, you wouldn't want to throw on all of your wood at once."

"No? Why not?" Mike asked.

"Because if you did that the fire would blaze madly for awhile and quickly burn up all the logs. Before morning, the fire would be out. On the other hand, if you took the same amount of wood and fed logs to the fire gradually during the night, in the morning you'd still have a nice warm fire. You might even have some logs left over.

"Eating to help control your diabetes is like feeding logs to that fire a few at a time. Distributing food throughout the day will keep the fire burning more evenly than if you ate just one or two big meals each day. That's why dividing the daily food into three meals and three snacks helps people with Type I diabetes maintain stable blood sugar control."

"But isn't it true that at certain times during the day my insulin is having a greater effect than it does at others? What should I do then?"

"When your insulin peaks, holding the door wide open and creating a draft to fan the flames, you need to put large logs (meals) on the fire. When you have less insulin on board and the door begins to close, only small logs (snacks) should be added.

"On your program of a split-dose of mixed insulins, you have four insulin peaks:

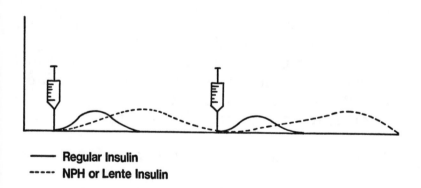

——— Regular Insulin
----- NPH or Lente Insulin

"So your three meals and bedtime snack will probably be larger than your morning and afternoon snacks. Different insulin regimens work best with different patterns of meals and snacks."

"But isn't that a lot of food? Three meals AND three snacks?"

The educator replied, "I'm not suggesting you eat more food each day. What I'm recommending is that you take the total amount of food that's right for you and divide it into three meals and three snacks. This will help produce better blood sugar control and protect you against low blood sugar reactions."

"I can see that. But I'm still puzzled about how much of different things I should eat," Mike responded. "Why is my blood sugar too low on an afternoon when I have a steak and salad for lunch instead of my usual sandwich? I know the steak has more calories than the sandwich."

The educator complimented the young man on his powers of observation and then explained. "The starches and sugars provided by carbohydrate-containing foods like the two pieces of bread in your usual sandwich are all converted to blood sugar. The steak's calories come from protein and fat, not from carbohydrate. Only a little more than half the calories from protein and less than 15% of the calories from fat end up as blood sugar.

"To balance your insulin and your meals, you need to be consistent with the servings of bread, cereal, pasta, milk, fruit and other carbohydrate foods. Having twice as much fruit as usual will make a much bigger difference in your blood sugar than having an extra pat of margarine or a larger-than-normal hamburger patty."

"So it matters what I eat. Does it matter when I eat too?" asked Mike.

"Yes, it really does. Have you heard that old saying, 'Timing is everything?'" the educator asked. "It sounds to me like whoever made that one up could have been talking about diabetes."

"I learned from the doctor to eat 45 to 60 minutes after I take my insulin. Is there anything else I need to know about timing?"

"Well, that's a great start," she answered, "but it's just one consideration. Waiting TOO long to eat can cause just as many problems as not waiting long enough.

"For example, some people delay eating when their blood sugar is too high before a meal. They keep testing until their insulin has brought the blood sugar down and then go ahead and eat the meal. This amounts to throwing a big log on the fire at the wrong time. It can lead to an upward swing in blood sugar because the big demand for insulin comes AFTER the strongest action of the insulin is past.

"Other people eat on time but make the mistake of varying their food intake based on their blood sugar."

"What do you mean?" Mike asked.

"Well, a person trying to manage blood sugar this way would decrease the size of the bedtime snack if blood sugar was above normal at that time. He or she might even skip it altogether if the sugar was quite elevated."

"Makes sense to me," the young man commented. "You wouldn't want to drive a high blood sugar even higher by eating, would you?"

"That sounds logical. But the problem is you might not have enough fuel to keep the fire going all night long if you skip the bedtime snack. Your chances for a low blood sugar reaction would be greater than if you'd eaten as usual."

"But doesn't having a high blood sugar at bedtime protect me from a middle-of-the-night reaction?"

"Not necessarily. Remember the overall goal is to match food peaks and insulin peaks. A blood sugar peak at bedtime doesn't match up with the peak of your insulin that acts overnight. That peak comes hours later. After all, 12 to 15 hours can go by between your evening meal and breakfast. That night snack is really important—even when your sugar is higher than you want it to be at bedtime."

"Gee, and I used to think the most important thing about my diet was to avoid sweets. It's definitely more complicated than that."

Nutrition in a Nutshell

1. A varied and healthful diet is the foundation of good diabetes control.

2. An adequate number of calories are needed to maintain normal weight and fuel your activity.

3. Delaying or skipping meals or snacks can cause problems.

4. Matching insulin and food curves allows for the most stable blood sugar control.

5. Food labels help you identify and avoid foods with a high sugar or fat content.

We can float among the stars together, you and I,
And we can fly.

The Fifth Dimension

CHAPTER 5

Installing the Altimeter: Monitoring

After the young man had mastered the basics of insulin and food, he and the educator concentrated on how to monitor his diabetes control. She told him they would be monitoring three different indicators of diabetes control, and two of these would be his responsibility.

"I know you've been doing finger-stick blood sugars for quite a while. Let's talk about ways to use them to get better control."

"I'll bet you've got another story," the young man observed.

"How did you guess?" she replied. "Controlling your diabetes is not only like riding a bike. In some respects it's also like flying an airplane. A pilot flying his plane at 5,000 feet checks his altimeter to determine whether he's maintaining the proper distance from the ground. And he doesn't just check his altimeter once during a trip. He checks it repeatedly, because a single reading could be misleading."

"What do you mean?"

"If he were to glance at his altimeter only once and it read 5,000 feet, he could assume he's flying straight and level at the desired altitude. But that single reading could also mean he was passing through 5,000 feet on his way up into the stratosphere. Worse yet, he could be diving through 5,000 feet, toward a close encounter of the painful kind with the ground.

"The pilot takes a series of altimeter readings in order to confirm that he is flying straight and level. Blood sugar readings work the same way. A single reading—whether low, normal or high—doesn't tell you all you need to know. To find out whether you're flying straight and level within your desired range of blood sugars, you have to take readings in sequence. Then you can see patterns emerge."

"So, what would you like me to do?"

"I recommend that you test four times each day—before meals and at bedtime. This will show us the trend of your blood sugar control throughout the day. You've told me before you'd like to keep your blood sugars near normal in order to feel your best and reduce your risk of complications. Our goal will be to have these readings fall between 80 and 140 milligrams per deciliter most of the time. Once your level of control stabilizes within this range, we'll know we've worked out the correct match among your insulin, food and exercise using Dynamic

Insulin Dosing. When that happens, you'll be able to cut back your blood testing schedule."

"Then I'll just be doing a test every couple of days?" asked Mike.

"No, we'll still ask you to test four times a day on the days you do test. Remember, four tests in one day allow us to see the pattern for the day.

"And keep in mind your blood sugars won't ALWAYS be in the target range, even when you've done everything 'by the book.' Having unexplained high blood sugars occasionally is just part of having diabetes. Our goal isn't perfection because it's just not possible. Our goal is to get the majority of your blood sugar readings in the target range the majority of the time. That's why we use blood sugar PATTERNS to adjust your insulin, instead of responding to a single high reading.

"Also remember there's no such thing as 'bad' blood sugar. Your blood sugar record only contains bits of information. It's not a moral score card. Every blood sugar reading you take the time, effort and expense to obtain is a 'good' blood sugar because it's a valuable piece of information. Whether it's above, below or within your target range, it's information you can act on to maintain or improve control over your diabetes.

"The second sort of test that would be helpful for you to do regularly is urine testing."

"Really?" asked the young man. "I thought urine testing was obsolete now that we do finger-stick blood sugars. I know for a fact urine sugar tests aren't very accurate."

"Urine tests for sugar really AREN'T very accurate as a means of inferring what your blood sugar is," the educator agreed. "But we recommend you test your urine, not just for sugar, but also for ketones." (See table on page 45 for help interpreting urine tests for sugar and ketones.)

"What's a ketone?"

"Ketones are a type of chemical that shows up in the urine when your diabetes is getting out of control. Blood sugar testing doesn't tell you whether you are producing ketones or not. Blood glucose meters aren't designed to detect them.

"That's why we recommend daily urine ketone testing for everyone who has Type I diabetes. We also recommend urine ketone testing during periods of illness for people who have Type II diabetes and take insulin. We'll talk in detail later about your action plan for days when you are ill. That's when I'll give you specific instructions on how to use urine ketone testing results. For now, all I want you to realize is that daily urine testing for sugar and ketones is part of our overall plan for monitoring your diabetes."

"OK, I can wait. But you said there was a third kind of test I should know about."

"That test is called a glycosylated hemoglobin. Years ago, the only tool a doctor had to evaluate how well someone's diabetes was being controlled was a fasting blood sugar. The doctor got one of these every few weeks or months. They had serious drawbacks."

"Really?"

"Yes, really. Their main weakness was how little information they gave the doctor. It was very difficult to make helpful adjustments in the insulin dose or recommended diet based on a single fasting blood sugar reading. And just as important, they couldn't give the doctor a clear picture of how well or poorly the management plan was working. There wasn't any way to know what the 'average' blood sugar had been from day to day since the last visit.

"And from the viewpoint of the person with diabetes, going into the doctor's office to have blood drawn for a fasting blood sugar was far from ideal. The best that could be expected was a hungry morning spent waiting in the doctor's office. And sometimes the doctor was delayed, adding to the difficulties. Most of the time, the patient's routine was badly upset. This happened because the person almost always waited to take his insulin until after the blood had been drawn AND he had seen the doctor. This would throw off the timing of meals and insulin for the rest of the day. And then the blood sugars would almost certainly go out of control."

"I know what you mean. I've been through it more than once."

"These days, self-monitoring of blood glucose provides a great deal more information. It's information that is especially valuable for managing day-to-day variations in food, insulin and activity. But each finger-stick blood sugar, just like a fasting blood sugar, only measures the blood sugar at one point in time.

"And you know blood sugars vary from hour to hour during the day. So self-monitoring still doesn't reveal a true average of recent blood sugar control."

"So what do we do?"

"Well, that's where the glycosylated hemoglobin test comes in. It allows us to see the *average* blood sugar level over the past several weeks."

"I know hemoglobin has something to do with the blood. But what in the world is *glycosylated*?"

"Picture one of your red blood cells as an apple. If we dipped the apple in sugar syrup, it would come out coated with a certain amount of sugar. The thicker the syrup, the thicker the coating of sugar on our candied apple," said the educator.

"Red blood cells have a lifespan of about 120 days. As they move around the body in the bloodstream, they pick up more or less 'sugar coating,' depending on the amount of sugar in the blood. That sugar-coating process is called *glycosylation*. This is going on every minute of every day.

"By taking a blood sample about every three months and sending it to the lab, we can, in a sense, check the amount of sugar coating on the candied apple. If there was a lot of sugar in the bloodstream during the last few weeks, the glycosylated hemoglobin will be above normal. If the average blood sugar level was in the target range, the glycosylated hemoglobin will be lower. Our goal is a reading as close to the normal range as possible."

"You mean the same reading as for a person who doesn't have diabetes?"

"Yes, or close to it."

"I have to ask. Do my red blood cells really look like candied apples after going through my bloodstream?"

"No, not really. But that's an easy way to make sense out of this test. What actually occurs is a chemical reaction. We just measure the result of that reaction to determine what your overall blood sugar control has been like."

Mike left the office that day thinking what a change it was to be working with people who listened to his questions. He really enjoyed having his questions answered in ways he could understand.

Monitoring

1. Finger-stick blood sugars before meals and at bedtime show your pattern of blood sugar control.

2. Patterns are more informative than any single blood sugar value.

3. Testing urine for sugar and ketones can provide helpful information.

4. Glycosylated hemoglobin helps reveal overall diabetes control.

Interpreting Morning Urine Tests
for Sugar and Ketones

Urine tests for sugar and ketones give additional information that is not available through blood sugar testing. Using the following chart, you can interpret the readings you get. It is based on testing the first urine passed in the morning. The interpretations are true for people who begin to show sugar in the urine when their blood sugar exceeds 180 mg/dl. This is the case for most people, but exceptions do occur.

Negative Sugar/Negative Ketones
Overnight blood sugar stayed between approximately 60 and 180. This is the goal.

Negative Sugar/Positive Ketones
Overnight blood sugar did not go over 180. Ketones indicate a low blood sugar reaction may have occurred.

Positive Sugar/Negative Ketones
Overnight blood sugar at some point went over approximately 180.

Positive Sugar/Positive Ketones
Overnight blood sugar at some point went over approximately 180. The ketones indicate your diabetes is getting out of control.

As the miller told his tale, her face—at first just ghostly—turned a whiter shade of pale.

Procol Harum

CHAPTER 6

When the Fire Goes Out: Hypoglycemia

Time passed. Mike's blood sugars were improving. They were lower than they had ever been since he developed diabetes—so much lower, in fact, that he was having frequent low blood sugar reactions. Mike was frustrated. If good control meant having reactions nearly every day, he wanted no part of it.

"I'm really sick of insulin reactions!" he complained to the doctor. "I feel so rotten when my sugar bottoms out that I'm tempted just to keep it on the high side. I never had reactions when my blood sugars were always well above normal. Now that I'm in tight control, I feel worse than ever."

"But you're not in tight control, Mike," the doctor explained. "Having frequent low blood sugar reactions means your diabetes is out of control—out of control on the low side. When we started working together, your diabetes was out of control on the high side. Your reactions are telling us that we overshot the mark. Let's look at how to solve this problem."

Continuing the story of the fire in the log cabin, the doctor explained how low blood sugar reactions occur. Recalling that insulin holds the cabin door open so wood can be brought in to feed the fire, the doctor asked Mike what would happen if the supply of wood ran out.

"Well, the fire would go out," he replied.

"And that's exactly what happens when there isn't enough food around when insulin is acting. The body's energy-producing fire goes out. The body recognizes this situation as a real threat. It tries to correct the problem by releasing certain chemicals called hormones to raise blood sugar: glucagon, epinephrine, growth hormone and others. Besides raising your blood sugar, they can cause a number of physical symptoms. The process can make you feel pretty bad.

"What kind of symptoms do you have when your blood sugar gets low?" the doctor asked.

"I usually get shaky and break out in a sweat," the young man answered. "But there have been times when I've gotten very disoriented and was kind of bumbling around."

The doctor pointed out the importance of each person recognizing and being on the alert for his or her own particular symptoms of a falling blood sugar level. "Symptoms can run the gamut from weakness and shakiness to headaches or tingling around the mouth and lips. In fact, low blood sugar reactions can mimic almost any symptom you can imagine. For example, stomachaches, dizziness and nervousness all can be caused by low blood sugar.

That's why it's a good idea to check your blood sugar anytime you're not feeling right. This will tell you for sure whether or not you're having a reaction."

The doctor continued, "The symptoms can become quite severe. When they cause you to be disoriented or to lose your coordination, it's a sign the brain isn't getting enough fuel. You might even pass out if a reaction this severe goes untreated."

"That's scary," Mike said.

"You're right about that. And the scariest part is how a reaction that severe could lead to a serious accident if it happened while you were swimming, biking, driving, climbing a ladder or doing something similar. Besides, repeated severe reactions can potentially cause brain damage. At the very least, they can make you feel awful. In the worst case, they can put you in real danger."

"What can I do about it?"

"Quite a bit, actually. The picture isn't at all bleak if you're realistic and act accordingly."

The doctor went on to assure the young man. "Most low blood sugar reactions can be prevented by applying what you know about how food, insulin and activity affect your blood sugar.

"Remember when we first met, I compared managing your diabetes with riding a two-wheel bike? Well, if you keep everything centered when you're riding the bike, you keep your balance and pedal along without any problems. But if you lean too far one way or the other, the bike tips over and you fall.

"It's the same with diabetes. Think of skipping a snack, delaying a meal or changing the time of your insulin injection like leaning too far over on the bike. All of these can produce curve mismatch—when insulin and food curves don't match—setting you up for a low blood sugar reaction."

"But what should I do if one DOES occur, Doc?" the young man inquired. "I usually feel terrible when it happens. And it seems to take so long before I begin to feel better. I almost always end up stuffing myself before I feel human again."

"In an insulin reaction, the fire has gone out. So the goal is to get that fire going again using something that burns fast and hot. It's like using newspapers or small twigs to start the fire in the cabin's fireplace. Foods that act like 'newspaper' provide sugar in a quickly digested form. Fruit juice, regular soda pop or a glucose gel product are best because they are liquids. You don't have to waste time chewing or sucking on them. But glucose tablets, hard candy and even fruit will do the job if liquids aren't available.

"Quick-acting sugars will get you feeling better faster than other foods, but they will only support the blood sugar for a short time—sort of like newspapers will help start the fire but won't keep it going for long. So, if the next meal is more than an hour away, you'll need to put a 'log' on the fire."

"What's a 'log?'" Mike asked.

"'Logs' are foods like peanut butter sandwiches, meat sandwiches or cheese and crackers. These foods combine carbohydrate with protein or fat. They have more calories than just fruit or juice and they release sugar into the bloodstream slowly. This can help prevent another insulin reaction before the time for your next meal rolls around."

"I usually just move up the time of my next meal. That gives me logs, right?"

"It gives you logs all right," the doctor agreed, "but not in the best way possible. Changing the time relationship between the regular meal and your insulin may increase your risk of having another reaction later on."

"What do you mean?"

"Let's say you usually eat supper at 6 p.m. But today at 4:30 you have an insulin reaction and decide to eat supper then because you're feeling low."

"I've done that."

"The problem comes a little later in the evening. On a normal day, you would have the food from your 6 p.m. supper matching up with the insulin you inject at about 5:15. But today you ate your supper at 4:30 because of the reaction. By the time your evening insulin begins to peak, your supper is digested and long gone. You're probably going to 'run out of gas' and have another reaction later that evening."

"I've done that too! So, I'll do better if I eat my meals at the usual times, but treat reactions with 'newspaper and logs?'"

"Right," the doctor agreed. "By the way, keep in

mind you won't always feel symptoms when your blood sugar is getting too low."

"I learned that the hard way. Last spring I had a reaction that came on without any warning. I literally didn't know what hit me until I woke up to find myself looking into the eyes of a paramedic," the young man revealed.

"That's what's called an *asymptomatic* reaction, meaning you didn't have any symptoms. This can happen when, for some reason, your body doesn't release the hormones we talked about earlier in response to a falling blood sugar level. This is more common in people whose blood sugars have been in poor control for many years, but as you know from your own experience, it can happen to other people as well.

"Because you can't always rely on getting symptoms when your blood sugar is too low, my advice is to treat any blood sugar of 70 mg per deciliter or less with 'newspapers and logs.'"

"Why do you pick 70?"

"Home blood glucose meters are only accurate to within 10 to 15% of the actual blood sugar value. They will get you 'in the ball park' but will not necessarily give you the exact value. For example, if we sent your blood sample to the lab and got back the exact blood sugar value of 100 mg/dl, your meter could show any value between 85 and 115 and still be functioning just fine."

"But, Doc, that's quite a spread."

"That's the best you can do with these machines."

"You've got to be kidding. That doesn't sound very good."

"It's good enough to keep control of your blood sugar. The alternative is to spend $35,000 on the kind of machine they have at the lab and carry it around with you in a moving van.

"Meters are great, but they're not perfect," the doctor went on. "So we just need to use what we know about how precise they are. For example, in the case of a finger-stick blood sugar reading of 70, the true blood sugar could actually be lower, as low as the high 50's. So rather than risk a crash, I recommend you treat any blood sugar of 70 or lower immediately—even if you feel just fine."

"Immediately? Even if I'm in the middle of doing something important, like trying to make it to a business appointment on time?"

"Yes. Begin treatment immediately—at the first sign of a reaction. The longer you wait before you start treatment, the worse it can get and the harder it can be to correct. Better to arrive a little late than to get there disoriented or not at all because of a severe reaction."

"You mean like the one I had when I passed out. Could I have done anything to save that visit from the paramedics?"

"Yes, that was definitely a severe reaction. In a case like that, glucagon could have been helpful."

"Glucagon?" Mike asked. "What's that?"

"It's a hormone—a 'chemical messenger'—like insulin. Insulin's message is 'move sugar out of the blood stream and into the cells.' Glucagon's message is 'move sugar out of the liver and into the bloodstream.' Once released from the liver, that sugar will circulate to the body's cells. Insulin will then allow it to enter the cells, and you will begin to wake up. This can take as long as 10 to 15 minutes.

"When you wake up, the glucagon treatment should be followed up with 'newspaper and logs.'"

The doctor then gave the young man a prescription for a GLUCAGON EMERGENCY KIT.* "Get this now, before you need it, and keep it in an accessible place at home and at work. Friends, family or co-workers with whom you spend a lot of time should learn how to use it. It needs to be mixed at the time of use and injected like insulin. The people around you are the ones you'll be relying on to use it if you should ever have another severe reaction."

"Thanks, Doc. I guess the bottom line is to take the meals and insulin on time to prevent reactions and prepare in advance for any low blood sugar reactions that might still occur."

"That's right, Mike. Do the things we've talked about and wear your diabetes identification at all times. It could save your life if you are ever found unconscious. While it's best to keep the bike balanced, it's still a smart idea to wear a helmet, just in case."

*Available from Eli Lilly and Company, Indianapolis, Indiana.

Treat Low Blood Sugars
with "Newspaper and Logs"

---

1. *IDENTIFY THE REACTION.*

- Be aware that any symptom might be caused by a low blood sugar.
- Know your own usual symptoms of low blood sugar.
- Do a finger-stick blood sugar if you're not sure.

2. *BEGIN TREATMENT IMMEDIATELY.*

- Delay allows the reaction to become more severe and harder to treat.
- Delay can result in unconsciousness.

3. *START THE FIRE WITH "NEWSPAPER."*

- Drink eight ounces (or more) of fruit juice or regular soda pop.

OR

- Eat two or three glucose tablets or one package of glucose gel.

- If none of the above is available, eat anything sweet.
- Eat the next meal or snack on time. Do not eat it early because of the reaction.

4. *KEEP THE FIRE GOING WITH "LOGS."*

- If the next meal or snack is less than an hour away, no "logs" are needed.

continued on next page

- If the next meal or snack is more than an hour away, TREAT AS ABOVE, then add a "log" to the fire.
- Logs are foods that provide carbohydrate, protein and fat, such as:
    - A meat, cheese or peanut butter sandwich
    - Crackers with cheese or peanut butter
    - A glass of milk.

5. *PREPARE IN ADVANCE FOR SEVERE REAC-TIONS RESULTING IN LOSS OF CONSCIOUSNESS.*

- Obtain a GLUCAGON EMERGENCY KIT.
- Instruct family and friends in its use.
- If you are found unconscious, they should inject the glucagon immediately.

6. *ALWAYS WEAR YOUR DIABETES IDENTIFICA-TION.*

*I got the rockin' pneumonia and
the boogie woogie flu.*
                    Huey "Piano" Smith and the Clowns

CHAPTER 7

Burning the Furniture:
Sick Days

The next few weeks passed uneventfully. Mike was finally beginning to feel he had control over his diabetes, instead of the other way around. He had a few low blood sugar reactions, but they were mild and he was prepared to treat them. He was absorbed in his daily activities at home and at work. And his blood sugars were right where he wanted them to be. Most were in the target range he and his doctor had agreed on. Life was going well. As he walked into the diabetes educator's office, he almost shouted out the good news.

"This is the best part of my job, Mike. It's great to see what a change you've made using the information we've talked about. I'm delighted you're so satisfied with the results, too.

"But our work's not over," she continued. "Now that you've learned to ride the bike on the straight and narrow, you're ready to prepare for the obstacles.

You need a plan for riding the bike when the weather turns bad—when you get sick."

"But I'm feeling fine," the young man protested. "Why do I need to think about getting sick now. I just want to enjoy this big improvement."

"I understand that," she replied. "But once you're sick, it's too late to do all you can. There are some preparations that can keep a garden-variety illness like the flu or a cold from destroying the diabetes control you've worked so hard to establish."

"OK, you win. I'm ready for another story. Am I going to ride the bike, go flying or return to the log cabin?"

"The log cabin. How about if I go with you this time and keep you company," she offered. "Let's pretend we're in the log cabin on a freezing winter's night. We're relaxing in front of the fire . . . talking about something other than diabetes."

"Well, at least we took a break."

"Yes, but the fire is dying down, and we've used up all the firewood you brought in earlier. So you head for the door to bring in more wood from outside. But there's been a fierce storm with sub-zero temperatures and the door is blocked by ice and snow. It won't budge."

"Things are going from bad to worse here! What else can go wrong?"

"You try the windows, but they're frozen shut too. The cabin is getting cold. The flames in the fireplace are sputtering."

"Sounds like a real crisis," Mike said. "What do we do now?"

"We've got to keep warm. We'll freeze if we let the fire go out. So there's only one thing left to do. We'll have to burn the furniture. And so we start to pitch it into the fireplace.

"Obviously, this isn't a perfect solution. The furniture has paint, varnish and stain on it. It's a different kind of wood than firewood. When it burns, it gives off choking black smoke. The wood from the woodpile gave off clean white smoke. But at least we'll stay warm until morning."

"Saved by cheap chairs and our own ingenuity!"

"You're really getting into this, Mike. But don't forget there's a point to the story. Think of the storm like an illness—a cold, the flu or an infection. More strength is needed to hold a door open when a stormy wind blows. In the same way, during an illness the cells of the body have a harder time holding open the cell doors that allow sugar to enter and be burned for energy.

"Without the fuel provided by sugar, the cell needs to find another way to keep its energy-producing fire going. So it 'burns the furniture.' In this case the furniture is the fat inside the cell. When fat is burned for energy without sugar being available to burn with it, ketones are produced. They're just as noticeable as the black smoke from burning the furniture in the cabin."

"I've been sick a few times since I've had diabetes. I've never seen the 'black smoke.'"

"That's probably because you weren't testing your urine for ketones every morning, as you do now. We have you test every day so you'll notice as soon as possible if you're 'burning the furniture.' If that happens, we need to bring it to a halt as soon as we can."

"Why do we need to stop it?" the young man wondered. "Most people probably have plenty of 'furniture' to burn."

"It's important because, just like the black smoke from burning the furniture in the cabin polluted the atmosphere, large amounts of ketones can be dangerous too. They will eventually make the whole body too acid. That combination of too much sugar building up in the bloodstream with ketones and excess acid is a life-threatening condition called diabetic ketoacidosis."

"I don't like the sound of 'life threatening' very much. So what should I do if I find I'm burning the furniture?"

"Here's a list of several things to do when you're sick," the educator answered. (See list at right.) "Let's start with your insulin."

"I know I have to take my insulin every day without fail. But shouldn't I reduce the dose when I'm sick and not able to eat as much as usual?" the young man asked.

"No, and that's a common mistake," she answered.

When You're Sick

1. Take at least your usual dose of insulin. **Cutting back or skipping a dose of insulin can cause significant problems when you're sick.** Add supplemental insulin as indicated.

2. Use "Food Substitutions for Sick Days" if you're unable to eat your usual meals.

3. Test a double-voided* urine sample for sugar and ketones four times per day at the times of your usual finger-stick blood sugar readings.

4. Report vomiting episodes to your doctor immediately.
   - Take medications to control vomiting or diarrhea as directed.
   - Consume extra fluids (small frequent sips).
   - Use broth or fruit drinks to replace minerals lost during vomiting and diarrhea.

5. Maintain contact with your doctor.

6. Know when your doctor wants you to call next.

7. Know how to reach your doctor, especially during non-office hours.

8. If your doctor is not available, report to the emergency room if your illness persists or worsens.

---

*See page 69 for a description of how to obtain a double-voided urine sample.

"Remember, when you're sick the storm is raging, making it harder for the doors to the cells to remain open. Sugar can begin to rise in the bloodstream because it can't get into the cells. Not only that, but when you're sick, a number of hormones released by the body can raise the blood sugar level even more."

"But how can that happen if I don't eat?" asked Mike.

"It happens because the liver can make sugar and release it into the bloodstream. And it makes and releases sugar at a much higher rate when we're sick than when we're well. It doesn't need food to do that. So even if you haven't eaten a thing, you might find your blood sugar getting higher."

"How do you stop the liver from doing that?"

"Insulin will slow down the sugar-producing factory in the liver and help bring things under control," she explained.

"I get it. Not taking insulin when you're sick can make matters worse by allowing the liver to make all that extra sugar."

"Exactly. That's why it's vital to always take at least your normal dose of insulin and never skip a dose, even when you're sick and can't eat. In fact, the doctor may advise you to supplement your usual dose with some extra Regular insulin. (See guidelines at right.)When the storm is raging, you may need extra insulin to keep the sugars under control and correct for ketones. But the most important thing to remember is to stay in close contact with the doctor's office whenever you're sick."

Supplements of Regular Insulin for Sick Days

Supplements of Regular insulin are taken for sudden temporary loss of diabetes control when you're ill. If your blood sugar is high when you're ill, add supplements before meals but not at bedtime. Do not supplement the bedtime dose because the extra insulin could cause a low blood sugar reaction during the night when you're sleeping.

Record all supplemental doses of insulin in your log book. If ketones are present, double the supplement and call your doctor. You should begin taking your supplements before your regular mealtimes as soon as you recognize that illness has disturbed your diabetes control. Do not take supplements at other times without consulting your doctor. The supplement is mixed with your usual insulin dose.

Supplements of Regular Insulin
(Do not take supplements at bedtime.)

For a blood sugar of . . .	Add
less than 200	0 units of Regular
200 to 249	1 unit of Regular
250 to 299	2 units of Regular
300 to 349	3 units of Regular
350 to 399	4 units of Regular
400 or more	5 units of Regular

**Double the supplement if ketones
are present in the urine.**

Note: Supplemental regular insulin is to be used only when you are ill. When you are well, make necessary insulin adjustments according to the Dynamic Insulin Dosing [SM] Guidelines.

Food Substitutions for Sick Days

When you're sick and not feeling well enough to eat as you normally do, it's still very important to take in adequate amounts of food and liquid. **Don't cut back on your dose of insulin or skip any injections, as this could lead to significant problems.**

If you're nauseated or your appetite is poor, it's not necessary to compensate for the fats or meat in the food you normally eat. On the other hand, it's very important that you take in enough carbohydrate to cover your insulin. *(Remember, insulin is like air. You must take it every day, even when you can't eat normally.)* When you're sick, try one of the following for each serving of starch, milk or fruit you normally eat:

1/2 cup apple, orange, grapefruit or pineapple juice
1/3 cup cranberry juice cocktail, grape juice or prune juice
3/4 cup regular (not sugar-free) soda pop
2 tsp. honey
2 1/2 tsp. sugar
1/3 cup regular (not sugar-free) JELL-O®
6 Lifesavers®
7 jelly beans
1/2 twin Popsicle®

1 slice bread or toast
6 saltine crackers
1/2 cup hot cereal
1/2 cup ice cream
1/2 cup sherbet

1 cup soup
1/3 cup tapioca or pudding
1 cup plain yogurt
1/2 cup commercial eggnog

In a nutshell, many of the foods you generally avoid when you're well are the ones to eat when you're sick!

"What about food?" inquired Mike.

"Well, you know from experience that you often don't feel like eating much when you're sick. Even the kinds of foods you want and can tolerate may change."

"So what should I do? I'm taking my insulin and I have to eat something, right?"

"True. Actually, when you're sick you can eat a lot of things you stay away from when you're well. Here's a list (at left) you should keep handy."

"But I've been told not to eat lots of these things because I have diabetes."

"You noticed that! And, of course, that's good advice when you're feeling well. But the fact that these foods have a large amount of sugar in a small amount of food is what makes them good choices when you're sick. Even when you don't feel like eating very much, you can eat small amounts of these foods and get enough calories to keep you going and balance your insulin."

"There's sure a lot to know about being sick."

"That's true," the educator agreed. "But it's worth the effort. Doing these things minimizes the effect a simple illness can have on your diabetes. And you may save yourself the expense of a stay in the hospital that could have been avoided."

Continuing through the "When You're Sick" list, the educator discussed the importance of drinking plenty of fluids during an illness. "It's easy to get dehydrated when you're sick—even easier when you have diabetes, too. You may not drink as much as usual because you're nauseated. You may lose extra fluids through vomiting or diarrhea. And if your blood sugar starts to get high, you'll lose even more water through the urine."

"But what if I'm really sick to my stomach and not able to keep much down?"

"Try swallowing small sips slowly. Take your time. It may take as long as a half hour to get down a half cup of fluid when you're sick. Doing it this way may help to 'sneak it' past an upset stomach. If you try to swallow a full glass all at once, you'll increase the chances of tossing it back up."

"Is there anything else I can do if I can't sneak it past my stomach?" asked Mike.

"Let's have the doctor write a prescription for a medicine to control nausea and vomiting. I recommend you fill the prescription today so you have the medicine on hand the next time you need it. If you're THAT sick, you won't feel like running out to the pharmacy to pick up supplies."

"That makes sense. Is there anything else I should keep around the house for the next time I get sick?"

"Yes. Keep the doctor's and the pharmacy's phone numbers handy. Get a thermometer so you can tell the doctor your temperature. Get some of those items from the *"Food Substitutions for Sick Days"* list. Also lay in a supply of nonprescription medicines that you can use when you're under the weather: things like cough medicine and pain relievers. Some of those products have a good deal of sugar in them, so I'll give you a list of medicines that are sugar-free and safer for you to use. (See page 68).

"How about testing," Mike inquired. "Should I test any differently when I'm sick?"

"Because things can change so quickly when you're sick, testing is even more important than when you're well. Do at least four blood sugar tests each day, and of course, test any time you think you might be having a low blood sugar reaction."

"How about urine testing? Is that any different when I'm sick?"

"Yes, it is. When you're sick, we recommend that you do a urine test four times a day, at about the same times you do your finger-stick blood sugars. In this way, you'll know right away if you start to burn the furniture. If that happens, call the doctor so he can help you stay right on top of the situation.

"I'd like you to use a *double-voided urine* sample for the ketone tests you do during an illness. Then you'll be able to tell if the body is still making ketones at the time you do the test. You can be confused by a first-voided urine sample because it might contain ketones produced some time before. They can still be there in the bladder if you haven't urinated in the last few hours, even though your body may have stopped ' burning the furniture' already."

"What do you mean by a 'double-voided' sample?"

Sugar-Free Non-Prescription Medicines

Some over-the-counter medicines, such as pain killers, cough medicines and antacids, contain sugar. The amounts are generally small and may not disturb your diabetes control. But since illness makes it more difficult to control your diabetes anyway, its best to choose sugar-free varieties when possible.

This list will help you choose over-the-counter medications that won't make it even harder to control your diabetes when you're feeling sick. It is helpful to: (1) Read labels on medications. Avoid those that contain sugar (sucrose, glucose, sorbitol, mannitol, fructose or dextrose) or alcohol. Read the label every time you buy one of these products because manufacturers occasionally change their formulations. (2) Test your blood sugar frequently when you're sick.

Cough Medicines (sugar-free, containing little or no alcohol)
Cerose-DM Liquid
Colrex Cough Syrup
Colrex Expectorant Syrup
Contac Jr. Liquid
Hytuss Tablets
Naldecon-DX
Scot-Tussin Syrup
Tolused-DM Liquid

Decongestants
Dimetane Decongestant Elixir
Dimetapp Elixir
Novahistine Elixir
Sinutab Maximum Strength Nighttime Liquid
Afrin Nasal Spray
Neo-Synephrine Nose Drops

Pain and Fever Medications (Avoid aspirin. Even though sugar-free, it raises blood sugar in large doses.)
Datril
Panadol
Tylenol
Generic acetaminophen
Nuprin
Generic ibuprofen
Children's Panadol (liquid, drops, tablets)
Dolanex Elixir

"To get a double-voided sample, empty your bladder but don't test that first sample. About a half hour later, urinate again. This is the sample you test. By doing this you get a more accurate reading of what the body is doing at the time of the test."

Mike left the educator and headed for home. On the way, he stopped at the pharmacy to pick up his sick day supplies. Then he went by the supermarket and stocked up on JELL-O, soda pop and Popsicles. As he stood in the candy aisle picking out a bag of jelly beans to keep around for sick days he thought to himself, "If my other docs could only see me now!"

Sick Day Summary

1. Keep a supply of sick day medications.

2. Use **Food Substitutions for Sick Days** to assure adequate calorie intake when you're too sick to eat your usual meals.

3. Drink plenty of fluids.

4. Take your temperature and record it daily while you're sick.

5. Keep the doctor's and pharmacy's phone numbers handy at all times.

6. Check and record blood sugar and urine ketones at least four times a day while you're sick.

7. Call the doctor if ketones are present.

SECTION II:

The Flashy Plays

Jeremiah was a bullfrog.
He was a good friend of mine.
I never understood a single word he said,
but I helped him drink his wine.

Three Dog Night

CHAPTER 8

Joy to the World: Entertaining

"I'm still not sure how I should handle eating out or going to parties," Mike told the educator at their next visit. "Whether I'm going out for fun or for business, those kinds of things almost never follow my usual schedule. Several times I've had pretty severe insulin reactions when dinner didn't arrive until after a long cocktail hour.

"It seem they always throw my timing off. You know I usually take my evening insulin at about a quarter to 6 and eat dinner around 6:30. Most of these things don't even start 'til 7, and that's usually just the cocktails. Dinner might not show up until 8 or sometimes even later."

"A change in meal timing after you've taken your insulin can create problems all right," the educator agreed. "Sometimes people who don't have diabetes have a hard time understanding that."

"Well, at least I've been able to come up with a comparison that my friends seem to understand. Now they listen up when I say it's time to get something to eat."

"What do you tell them?"

"Well, I tell them food to me is like air to a scuba diver. A given amount of air in a tank lasts only so long, and then it's time to get another tank. Then I tell them, 'Pretend you're going diving. Your tank has exactly enough air for one hour. How important would time be to you if you were trapped on the bottom and I promised to bring you a new tank . . . in an hour and ten minutes?'"

"That's a great comparison. Can I use that example with my other patients?"

"Be my guest," the young man replied. "But first help me figure out how to handle my food and insulin so eating out and going to parties aren't such big problems."

"Well, I think the troubles you mentioned are probably related to both delayed meals and to drinking alcohol. If we discuss some ways to handle both kinds of situations, I think we'll solve your low blood sugar problems," the educator observed.

She then went on to explain that there are at least two ways of dealing with delayed meals. One is used when the meal is expected to be only an hour or so later than usual. In that case, simply delaying the time of the insulin injection by an hour will solve the timing dilemma.

"It will probably be helpful to add a small snack—the equivalent of a fruit or starch exchange—at about your usual meal time. Otherwise the insulin from your previous injection may drop your blood sugar too low before you eat."

"But the delays are usually a lot longer than an hour when I eat out with friends or for business."

"Yes, those 8 or 9 o'clock suppers are an entirely different matter," advised the educator. "We have a different way to manage those.

"When you're expecting a late supper, take your pre-dinner insulin injection at the usual time. Then move the amount of food that is in your usual bedtime snack into the time slot when you usually have your supper. Depending on the kind of evening you have planned, you might have that snack before you leave home.

"But if there's a cocktail hour, it will make more sense to eat your snack during cocktails. There are usually hors d'oeuvres available. Some combination of crackers, cheese, vegetables and fruit that approximates your usual bedtime snack should work well. Be sure to get about the same amounts of carbohydrate foods—the starches and sugars provided by bread, fruit and milk—since this is what will protect you from a low blood sugar reaction. If food is not available, use fruit juice or regular soda pop as a drink or mixer."

"What about the dinner?"

"When dinner finally arrives, just stay as close to your normal meal pattern as possible. This whole system works because you're taking in approximately the same total amount of food relative to the same total amount of insulin. It's like depositing your paycheck on the first of the month but waiting until the fifteenth to pay your bills because you've been out of town. The checkbook balance at the end of the month is the same as if you had paid your bills on the first."

"But if I'm going to have a drink during the cocktail hour, shouldn't I decrease the size of my snack? I've got an exchange list for alcohol at home."

"Exchanging alcohol for food is an important concept for people with Type II diabetes who don't take insulin and are trying to lose weight. The high calorie content of alcohol is their main concern. But when you're taking insulin, especially if you have Type I diabetes, the approach is different.

"Most people don't realize that pure alcohol alone doesn't raise blood sugar. In fact, if taken on an empty stomach when you have insulin on board, it can cause a severe low blood sugar reaction. That's why it's important to eat if you're going to be drinking alcohol."

"So that's where those reactions have been coming from. I've always reduced the size of my meal when I had a cocktail or two before dinner."

"Well, now you know how to handle it, Mike. But one last thought. If you're going to drink alcohol, keep the amounts moderate—no more than one or two drinks in a day. More alcohol can really interfere with the control you've been working so hard to establish."

"You know," said the young man, "some of these parties go on for hours. Two drinks won't go very far. But I guess I could switch to diet soda or sparkling water after I reach my limit."

"That's a great idea," she congratulated him. "You know, if your friends are like mine, they're probably so absorbed talking shop or having a good time that they don't really care what you're drinking anyway. The important thing is for you to find a comfortable way to participate fully, without creating a big change in the control of your diabetes."

Alcohol, Insulin and Type I Diabetes*

1. If you drink, limit it to two drinks per day.

2. Your best choices are distilled liquor (vodka, gin, bourbon, etc.) with non-caloric mixers, dry wines and light beers.

3. Eat your usual amount of food. Drinking on an empty stomach can result in severe low blood sugar reactions.

4. If possible, make sure someone in the group knows you have diabetes and how to treat a low blood sugar reaction.

5. Gasoline and alcohol don't mix. Make sure there's a designated driver in your group.

* If you have Type II diabetes and are overweight, use exchanges to fit alcoholic beverages into your meal plan. If you have Type II diabetes, are normal weight and take insulin, follow the guidelines given here for Type I diabetes.

Out on Runway Number Nine, big 707 set to go,
But I'm stuck here on the grass
where the pavement never grows.

Peter, Paul and Mary

CHAPTER 9

The Road to Zanzibar: Travel

"Doc," Mike said some weeks later, "I'd like to start planning for my vacation. Do you have any advice?"

"Well, first of all, travel, like the rest of life, can be a lot of fun. But it can also be trying and frustrating.

"As you make your travel plans, keep Murphy's Law in mind: 'Anything that can go wrong will.' Applied to your vacation, Mike, that means travel is made fun and less stressful by anticipating the snafu's that might occur. Then you can preempt them with planning. The unexpected will still happen—but you'll be ready for it.

"The most important thing to remember is that without your insulin, your vacation would come to an abrupt end. If you break your last bottle of insulin at home, you know exactly where to go to get more in a hurry. Away from home, it wouldn't be that simple."

As the two discussed how to prepare for his coming vacation, the young man began to understand the importance of bringing a back-up supply of insulin on every trip. The doctor also explained the value of carrying the bottles in current use separately from the extras. The young man also learned to keep all insulin in hand-carried bags, since luggage compartments and car trunks may reach temperatures (both too hot and too cold) that can reduce insulin's effectiveness.

"But what if somebody walks off with my carry-on bags?" Mike asked.

"Good for you. Now you're thinking like Murphy himself! I'll give you prescriptions for your insulin, syringes and a GLUCAGON EMERGENCY KIT. Keep them in your wallet or passport case. They could save the day in a real pinch."

"Will I need to change my insulin dose to make a trip?" the young man inquired.

"If you're traveling more than two hours out of our local time zone, you'll need to adjust the amounts and timing of your insulin doses. When you know your destination and your travel schedule, we can work out a transition plan. That plan will be based on whether you're traveling east or west and how many hours difference there is between home and your vacation spot."*

"How about if I limit all my vacations to places either north or south of here, instead of east or west? Then we wouldn't need to adjust the insulin."

*See *Insulin Adjustments for Time Zone Changes*, page 85.

"Well, that's an idea, isn't it?" chuckled the doctor.

"An idea, just not a great one. Wherever I do decide to go, I'll probably be going by plane," the young man said. "What can go wrong?"

"Just about everything," the doctor answered. "ASSUME that planes will be late, meals will be absent or delayed, checked luggage will be lost. Carry all the diabetes supplies you might need right on you.

"Don't check anything you can't afford to be without. And never carry more than you can comfortably schlepp across Chicago-O'Hare at a full gallop when you end up with only 30 minutes between planes. At the very least, carry insulin, syringes, testing supplies and food to last a day. Carrying glucagon is a good idea, too, especially if you'll be traveling with someone whom you've taught to use it.

"If you'll be taking an insulin injection during your flight, you won't need to inject air into the bottle before drawing up the dose. The cabin pressure at high altitudes on commercial airliners will take the place of injecting air into the vial."

"How about eating on the plane?" asked the young man.

"Airline 'diabetic' meals may be more trouble than they're worth. They run the gamut from something remarkably like the 'regular' meal (except for the fact the flight attendant walks up and down the aisle with yours yelling 'Who's got the diabetic meal?') to the thoroughly ridiculous 'super diet' meal that may not have enough calories to cover your normal insulin dose.

"Our educator recommends you take your chances with the regular meal, supplementing or substituting from your own food supplies as necessary to match your normal meal pattern. You can usually count on being able to get both regular and diet soda as well as fruit juice on flights lasting longer than 45 minutes.

"And finally, walk around frequently during long flights and drink plenty of extra fluids. The air is much drier at high altitudes. If you just sit there during the flight, much less active than usual, your blood sugar may tend to rise. You know from experience that you urinate more when your blood sugar is high. The dry air, a high blood sugar and frequent urination working together can make you quite dehydrated. But if you remember to drink enough liquids and move around occasionally, you'll arrive feeling much more energetic!"

"What if I decide to go on that European vacation you mentioned on our first visit?" asked the young man.

"Sounds great to me," answered the doctor. "But there are a few extra things to keep in mind. Probably most importantly, different types and strengths of insulin are sold in other countries, compared with what you're using here. Since any change in the type, brand or source of insulin you're using is likely to require you to adjust your doses to maintain blood sugar control, it's best to take extra insulin with you. If you must make a change in your type of insulin while on a trip, test your blood sugar more frequently and use Dynamic Insulin Dosing to get the dose stabilized as quickly as possible.

"Remember that water supplies and standards of sanitation may be different from what you're used to here at home. Exotic 'bugs' in food and water could bother you. If you decide on a trip outside the country, you might find our list of *Travel Tips* helpful. (See page 88).

"Once you know what to do about the safety of the food you'll be eating. there's another challenge in store for you. That challenge is to create a reasonable equation between the unfamiliar foods being served and the usual meals you eat here at home. When you decide on your destination, ask our educator for the food exchange list for the foods of the country you'll be visiting. Food exchange lists are available for many different countries. After all, we're not the only place in the world that has diabetes.

"Even though you're not using an exchange meal plan yourself just now, you can study the lists to familiarize yourself with the foods you'll encounter on your trip. It will also help you identify serving sizes that match up with the way you eat at home.

"Finally, before leaving home, do some research and prepare a contingency plan to obtain medical care while on an international trip. One way to begin is to contact the International Association of Medical Assistance to Travelers.* If language will be a

---

*International Association of Medical Assistance to Travelers, 736 Center Street, Lewiston, New York 14092.

barrier, also be sure to learn at least the phrases you would need to obtain medical services and order appropriate meals."

"All this preparation sounds more like planning a military campaign than heading off on a vacation."

"Yes, there really is quite a bit to consider. But if you take care of all the details, Mike, you should be able to travel anywhere your bank account will allow."

Insulin Adjustments for Time Zone Changes

It is necessary to adjust your insulin when traveling more than two time zones to the east or west. Here are two of the most common ways this type of adjustment can be made.

Option 1.

Switch to a "Basal/Bolus" insulin regimen well before your trip. Basal/bolus therapy involves taking a dose of regular insulin about 45 minutes before each meal (a "bolus) and one or two doses of long-acting insulin to provide a small steady amount of insulin all day and night (the "basal").

• **If traveling west to east** so your day is shortened by three or more hours, decrease the basal insulin acting on the day you travel by 20%.

• **If traveling east to west** so your day is lengthened, add a bolus of Regular insulin for any additional meal(s) eaten on the travel day.

Option 2.

**•Traveling West to East
(Day shortened by three or more hours.)**

One injection per day—Decrease dose by 20% on your travel day. Re-establish your regular schedule on the first full day at your destination. Get up on "their" time and proceed with your usual meal and insulin schedule.

Split dose—Decrease the second dose by 20%. All 20% can be taken off the NPH or Lente unless you will be eating a much lighter dinner than usual in deference to the time change. In that case, divide the reduction between the short-acting and the inter-mediate-acting insulins. Re-establish your regular schedule on the first full day at your destination. Get up on "their" time and proceed with your usual meal and insulin schedule.

**•Traveling East to West
(Day lengthened by three or more hours.)**

One injection per day—Increase your dose by 10% on your travel day.

Two injections per day—Add a bolus of regular insulin equal to about 10 to 15% of your total daily dose before the extra meal you eat on your travel day.

When You Travel

1. In a hand carried bag, pack:
   - at least one day's supply of food
   - insulin and syringes
   - glucagon
   - glucose meter, strips and lancets
   - urine ketone test strips
   - prescriptions
   - other medications you use
   - list of medical care facilities at destination.

2. Take a back-up supply of critical items, packed in a separate bag.

3. When crossing time zones, work out a transition plan for insulin with your doctor.

4. Before leaving home, prepare a plan for obtaining emergency medical care while you are away.

Travel Tips for Outside of North America

1. If safety of the local water supply is in question:
   - Drink bottled water. Carbonated beverages, beer and wine in bottles also are safe.
   - Don't use ice cubes.
   - Avoid foods that are washed and served without cooking, such as salad greens or raw fruits. Peeled fruits are ok.
   - Use dental floss to clean your teeth instead of tooth paste and water.

2. If food storage and preparation methods are unknown, in question or "non-western":
   - Eat hot foods hot and cold foods cold.
   - Foods containing mayonnaise are a risk if refrigeration is poor.
   - Raw meat and fish are a risk because they may carry parasites.
   - Dairy products, including milk and ice cream, are a risk because of lack of pasteurization in many countries.

3. Bring an adequate supply of personal toilet articles not always available outside of North America: facial tissues, soft toilet paper, and sanitary napkins.

4. In addition to insulin and your prescription medication, bring supplies you will need if you should become ill on your trip:
   - medication for nausea and vomiting
   - medication for fever and pain
   - medication for diarrhea
   - a thermometer

5. Bring generous amounts of diabetes supplies:
   - Urine strips for glucose and ketones
   - Finger-stick blood sugar strips
   - An extra blood glucose meter (Repair or replacement may be difficult.)
   - Extra batteries for your meter
   - Syringes

6. Know where to go for medical care. Get this information BEFORE leaving home.
   - If an emergency arises and you cannot reach the health care providers you have identified, contact the nearest Embassy or Consulate.

Let's get physical . . .

Olivia Newton-John

CHAPTER 10

Up Off the Couch!
Exercise

"You know, Doc," the young man observed, "there's something else I'd like to learn about—exercise. I love to run and play tennis. But in the past I've had such problems with low blood sugar reactions when I exercised that it didn't seem worth the trouble. It took all the fun out of it for me."

"Well, if it's not fun you probably won't do it. So let's see what we can do to help you enjoy it.

"First, it's great that you love to exercise. But, you know, there are some other good reasons to exercise BESIDES fun. Doctors have actually been recommending exercise for people with diabetes since about 600 B.C.

"People who exercise regularly have a greater sense of well-being and are better able to deal with stress. Their energy level is higher; their stamina is greater. Exercise even helps to lower blood pressure, control weight and decrease the risk for heart disease."

"I've heard all that before, Doc, but are the benefits worth the risk of a low blood sugar?"

"Yes, I think they are. Especially if you prepare. When you plan adequately, you greatly reduce the risk of reactions and other potential problems. But there are a few things you need to learn."

"So teach me! That's why I'm here."

"Well, the first step is picking your sport."

"I've heard lifting weights is not a good choice when you've got diabetes. Is that true?" the young man inquired.

"Yes, under certain circumstances," the doctor replied. "Weight lifting causes blood pressure to rise. The heavier the weight, the higher the pressure. This could be harmful to someone who has eye problems associated with their diabetes. It's also an issue with contact sports like football: further eye damage could be caused by a really hard tackle."

"Actually, I'd like to go back to jogging."

"That's a good choice for you. You don't have any joint or foot problems that might be stirred up by the impact of running. For people who do have those difficulties, walking and swimming would be better ways to get started. But now that you've picked your sport, let's prepare for it. I would recommend you start by getting good, well-fitting foot wear as well as good, well-fitting diabetes gear."

"Well-fitting diabetes gear?"

"Yes. For example, diabetes ID of some type—a bracelet or a neck chain—fits your needs. It can alert others to provide appropriate help if you should encounter any problems while exercising. And having a GLUCAGON EMERGENCY KIT along with other items to treat or prevent low blood sugar such as juice, crackers or glucose gel is also important. Of course, if you're planning long workouts, you'll need a supply of water. And it's best to have blood sugar testing materials with you as well."

"Are you sure you're not sending me out for an overnight camping trip, Doc? Where am I supposed to put all this stuff? I'd need to borrow the side-car off my brother's motorcycle."

"It's not that bad, Mike," the doctor laughed. "It will all fit in the same athletic bag you carry your sweats or shoes in. Most people just set the bag down in the area where they're working out."

"But how about when I run? If I'm two miles out and start to have a reaction, I'm not going to be able to make it back to some bag."

"For mobile exercise like running or biking, I'd recommend one of the 'runner's belts.' They have a good-sized compartment in them."

"My blood glucose meter won't fit in one of those. And I wouldn't want something that heavy jarring against me when I run anyway. I suppose I could just carry visually read strips and lancets. That's the way I used to test my blood before I got my meter."

"That's one solution," the doctor agreed. "Another possibility is one of the new, smaller meters. I think you'll be surprised by the selection. There are meters out there now no larger than a ball point pen or even a credit card. Remember, well-fitting gear gets the job done."

"I understand this is all stuff I would need in case something went wrong. But what I really want to know is how to keep it from going wrong in the first place."

"Thinking like Murphy again! You're OK," the doctor complimented him. "Actually I was just getting to that.

"The first way to avoid trouble is to make sure your diabetes is in adequate control before you begin to exercise."

"I know that. I always check my blood sugar before any kind of workout. If it's too high, I skip the exercise."

"But do you also check for ketones before you exercise?" the doctor asked.

"Ketones? No. Why?"

"A high blood sugar reading by itself may not necessarily be a reason to cancel a workout. Whether or not you have ketones in your urine is much more critical to your body's response to exercise. Just like you, a lot of people neglect that important step of checking for ketones.

"Remember the log cabin? When a positive test for ketones tells you you're 'burning the furniture,' you need to find out what the problem is and correct it before you begin to exercise. Otherwise, the exercise might just make matters worse."

"How can that happen?"

"Recall that you 'burn the furniture'—use fat for energy' -when blood sugar can't get into the cell where it's needed. This can happen when there isn't enough insulin around to keep the cell door open so sugar can get inside. Or it can happen when there just isn't any blood sugar available—like when you are having an insulin reaction.

"Since exercise increases the rate at which your body uses energy, exercising when ketones are present just makes you 'burn the furniture' at an even higher rate. In an extreme situation, all the ketones being produced could drastically change the chemical balance of the body and cause you to go into diabetic ketoacidosis."

"So, obviously, exercising when I'm positive for ketones would not be smart. What should I do?"

"If you find ketones when you get up in the morning and your blood sugar is in the normal or low range, test for ketones again a couple of hours after breakfast. If the ketones have disappeared, they were probably the result of a low blood sugar reaction during the night. You could go ahead with your exercise.

"If, instead, you find ketones and a fairly high blood sugar, say over 250, switch over to sick day procedures. Skip workouts until you're well and your diabetes is back in control."

"What should I do if my blood sugar is over 250 but I don't have any urine ketones?"

"If you feel good, go ahead and exercise. If you don't feel good, skip it. Just don't fall into the trap of feeling like you have to go out and exercise to bring down a blood sugar that's higher than you want it to be. Exercise for fun. Exercise for relaxation. Exercise for health. Use all the other tools we've talked about to keep your blood sugars where you want them to be.

"Right now, though, your main concern is low blood sugar reactions during exercise. So let me explain how exercise decreases your need for insulin.

"Let's go back to the log cabin again. If a stiff breeze began to blow, fanning the flames in the fireplace, the fire would burn much faster than before. You would have to feed logs to the fire at a faster rate. Exercise is like that stiff breeze. It causes you to burn fuel faster. It decreases your need for insulin. Think of it as a draft helping to keep the cabin door open and fanning the fire. So you need less insulin when you exercise."

"How much less?" he asked.

"That depends on how long and how vigorously you exercise. By monitoring your blood sugar before and after exercise, you can figure out how much to decrease the insulin. The reduction might be as little as 10% off for a one-hour run or as much as an 80 or 90% drop if you were going to run a marathon. If you're planning to exercise for less than an hour, eating an extra serving of fruit or starch will often work better than trying to make a very tiny insulin adjustment.

"By doing about the same amount of activity at about the same time each day, you can more easily adjust your insulin to that routine. If your exercise pattern is random, with workouts occurring at different times on different days, it is much trickier to make accurate insulin adjustments."

"When I was running regularly, it was nearly always in the morning. I'll probably do the same again. But how about times when I haven't planned on exercising? My girl friend likes to play tennis. But I usually don't know until the afternoon if we're actually going to play that day or not."

"For spur-of-the-moment increases in activity it's obviously too late to decrease insulin that was already injected earlier in the day. But even though you can't adjust the amount of insulin that's on board, you can adjust the amount of food that's available. The equivalent of a fruit or starch exchange for each 30 to 45 minutes of moderate intensity exercise should do the trick. You'll do better if you make this adjustment before and during exercise to PREVENT the onset of reactions instead of waiting to feel symptoms and then treating them."

"Sounds great. What kind of fruit or starch would you recommend?"

"Try whatever you enjoy that agrees with you when you're active. A half dozen soda crackers, a small box of raisins or a small can of orange juice can all work well and are pretty easy to carry in your bag of goodies. If your workout is going to be really lengthy, I'd concentrate on juices or soft fruits that provide fluids along with the carbohydrate."

"Is there anything else I need to do?" The young man was anxious to get started.

"Yes, as a matter of fact, there are two more things to be aware of. One is to make sure you get enough fluids when you exercise. Dehydration will jeopardize your athletic performance and can disturb your diabetes control as well.

"The last consideration is to make sure you get enough food—not only before and during your workout, but after it as well."

"What do you mean?" the young man asked.

"When you exercise for very long, your body uses up stored supplies of energy in the muscles and liver. It will replace these stores at some later time, after you've finished exercising. Your blood sugar is likely to drop quite a bit when that happens. So it's important to continue to monitor your blood sugar AFTER long workouts. An extra snack may be needed to prevent that drop in blood sugar. If you exercise late in the day, keep in mind that blood sugar could fall during the night.

"A long workout is sort of like taking out an energy loan from the bank. At some point you're going to need to pay it back. Make sure your body has something around to pay that blood sugar 'bill' when it comes due."

Getting Set to Exercise

Before you get started . . .

1. Obtain and wear a diabetes ID that shows your name, address, phone number, person to contact in an emergency and your doctor's name and phone number.

2. Invest in a well-fitting pair of good athletic shoes that protect and support your feet. If you have trouble getting a good fit, consult a podiatrist or an orthopedic specialist.

3. Get a GLUCAGON EMERGENCY KIT. Teach your running partner(s) how and when to use it.

4. Get a "runner's belt" to carry diabetes supplies.

What to take with you whenever you exercise:

1. Something to treat or prevent hypoglycemia:

-Glucose gel or tablets
-Candy
-Fruit juice or sport drink
-Fruit or crackers

2. Diabetes ID

3. Glucagon

For endurance events, also carry . . .

1. Water, if not available along your route.

2. Visual glucose strips, lancets, and watch or compact meter and supplies.

During exercise . . .

1. Check blood sugar and urine ketones before you begin.

2. Schedule workouts for the same time each day.

3. Drink plenty of fluids.

4. Eat enough food to fuel activity and cover your insulin.

I would not be convicted by a jury of my peers, still crazy after all these years.

Paul Simon

CHAPTER 11

Morley Safer's in the Waiting Room: Stress

The diabetes educator was reviewing the young man's blood sugar records at one of his periodic visits. She called his attention to a definite change in blood sugar patterns that occurred toward the end of each month.

"If you were a woman, I'd have a good idea of what's going on," the educator said. "For a lot of women, hormone changes during the menstrual cycle cause blood sugars to go out of control in a fairly predictable fashion. Changes in the insulin dose can usually compensate for that. But that can't be your problem can it, Mike? So what's up?"

"I've noticed the pattern myself," the young man replied. "The only thing I can think of is that I work longer hours toward the end of each month. I have to get all of my end-of-the-month paper work out."

"Maybe stress is having an effect on your blood sugar."

"Stress. I think you may be right," he replied. "Especially when I'm sitting there waiting for the sales figures to come in. My commission check depends on meeting those sales quotas."

"Well, I think we may have our answer," she agreed and went on to describe one way stress can disturb blood sugar control. She used Mike's hectic month-end schedule to illustrate her point. "By making demands on your time and your concentration, stress can affect your blood sugar by changing your routine. When you're feeling stressed you may not be as careful about keeping a consistent time relationship between your insulin and your meals. Or maybe you eat differently because you're rushed and don't take the time to prepare your usual meals.

"Some people use more sweets and alcohol during stressful periods. You might even get careless about how much insulin you're drawing up because you're worried about what the boss is going to think of your report. In short, there are a lot of ways feeling stressed can directly affect the way you manage your diabetes."

"I can see that, and I'm sure that was happening at first," said the young man. "But recently, I've been very careful about food and exercise. Even so, the blood sugars are still a little higher and more erratic during the last week of each month than they are at other times."

The educator then described the other way feeling stressed can affect blood sugar.

She explained that when life events are perceived as threats or "stressors," the body produces hormones that make fuel—sugar—more readily available in case a person needs to fight or run away. That was a great response when the threats people encountered were physical—a saber-toothed tiger waiting in the bushes or a neighboring tribesman charging up behind you, club in hand.

"Most of the things people think of as being stressful these days—a demanding supervisor, a quarrelsome neighbor, or snarled traffic—can't be dealt with in physical terms. And so the extra fuel made available by the stress response goes unused. In the person with diabetes, this creates a situation in which the usual insulin dose just can't keep things in line. This can lead to high or erratic blood sugars in response to stress.

"Stress is inevitable. Even good things like getting a promotion or buying a beautiful new car are potentially stressful. In fact, being ALIVE means you are subject to stress. But it's how we respond to potentially stressful changes and challenges that actually determines our level of stress. 'Stressors' are usually external events (although our own thoughts can certainly be stress-inducing), but 'stress' itself is always an entirely INTERNAL event."

The educator used a story to illustrate:

It's Friday night in Hoboken. Old Overshoe Airlines has the last flight of the evening to Chicago. The plane is an hour late and at least 50% overbooked. After the ticket agents calm down most of the crowd by giving them free tickets, two businessmen are left standing at the gate.

When informed he won't be able to get out of town until the "red eye" flight at 1 a.m., Fred B. Cool thanks the attendant, calls his wife, and sits down in the departure lounge with the latest adventure novel.

Frank Lee Steamed, on the other hand, makes a loud and detailed commentary on the ticket agent's IQ and threatens never to fly Old Overshoe again. He spends the next four hours reliving the entire experience in vivid color for everyone unfortunate enough to be within earshot.

"Frank is definitely having a stress reaction! But Fred accepts the change in plans with composure. He even uses the extra time to relax and enjoy himself. The external event is the same. It is what Fred and Frank are saying to themselves INTERNALLY that makes the event stressful or not.

"The message," said the educator, "is that things— both good and bad—that can lead to stress are bound to happen. When they do, your diabetes control may be affected. But you can reduce the negative impact of stress.

"Everybody has stress. It's one way of telling we're really alive. But some people seem to deal more effectively with it than others. You can minimize the effect of stress on your life, even though you can't make stress go away. You can ACT on your stressors, instead of letting them act on you."

Stress

1. RECOGNIZE when you're under excess stress.

2. EXAMINE what you are saying to yourself that makes events in your life seem more stressful.

3. COMMUNICATE your feelings openly to people whose actions add to your stress. Be assertive.

4. ACT to meet the challenge. Plan your time, manage your work and other demands.

5. MINIMIZE the effects of stress:
   • Approach life with a sense of humor—LAUGH!
   • Gain control of your life.
   • Make your life meaningful. Seek a defined role in family, work and community.
   • Approach life vigorously, seeing change as a challenge or opportunity.
   • Relax without guilt. Take time for leisure.
   • Attend to your physical needs through exercise and healthful food choices.
   • Get enough sleep
   • Limit or eliminate alcohol.
   • Abstain from using tobacco and other forms of substance abuse.
   • Work to develop a sense of inner security by identifying your values and priorities and acting in accordance with them.
   • Know how and when to practice some form of relaxation therapy, such as deep breathing or yoga.

Sweet dreams and flying machines in pieces on the ground.

James Taylor

CHAPTER 12

What Can We Learn from the Black Box? Research

"You know, Doc, my sister is worried she might get diabetes like I did."

"It's not an infection, Mike. She can't catch it from you."

"Oh, she knows that, but she's worried because we have diabetes in the family. She thinks she's sure to get it too. She even borrows my meter once in a while to test her blood sugar, to make sure she doesn't have it yet."

"That's understandable. It's a very common worry in the families of people who have diabetes. Brothers and sisters worry they'll get the disease. Parents worry their other children will develop diabetes. And the people who actually have it worry about whether they should have children for fear their kids may end up with diabetes too. So your sister's not alone in her concerns.

"But tell her there's a better test than a finger-stick blood sugar to let her know what's going on."

"What test is that?"

"It's called an *islet-cell antibody test.*"

"How does it work?"

"Well, Mike, we've talked about the fact you developed Type I diabetes because the beta cells in your pancreas were destroyed. We know the body's own immune system is involved in this somehow. But we don't know yet exactly what happens.

"When the immune system is destroying the beta cells, something called the islet-cell antibody shows up in the bloodstream. The antibody can be detected long before the blood sugar level shoots up. That's one of the reasons it's a better test for your sister than a finger-stick blood sugar. The presence of the islet-cell antibody in the bloodstream is an early marker for developing Type I diabetes. There are probably others, and research is being done to identify them. But the islet-cell antibody test is the first test of its kind to be made widely available."

"So this test can tell years in advance if someone is likely to get diabetes?'

"Right."

"That sounds like a really depressing piece of news to me. What possible good can come out of knowing for years that you're going to end up taking insulin and testing your blood someday?"

"I'm sure it sounds that way at first, Mike. But it's actually critical information. It's important, not only to the person who has the test done but also to everyone who might develop Type I diabetes in the future. That islet-cell antibody test is like the flight data recorder on a commercial airliner—that thing they call the 'Black Box.'"

"Doc, you two sure have a lot of stories about flying and airplanes. Are you a frustrated pilot?"

"Well, now you know my secret, Mike. But let me explain what I mean. When an airplane goes down, a team of investigators converges on the crash site searching for clues. Their goal is to prevent future crashes by learning what led to the specific crash they're studying. Their first job is to find the Black Box. Everything that happened in the final moments of the flight is recorded in that box. Using that information to reconstruct the flight and the crash, they can often pinpoint the exact cause of the crackup and even tell what might have been done differently to prevent it."

"So you're saying the beta cells of a person who will eventually develop Type I diabetes are like a plane headed for a crash?"

"Yes, in a way, they are. And researchers hope by improving our knowledge of what happens as diabetes develops, we'll also learn to treat it more effectively. We may even figure out how to prevent it in the future."

"Now that information would really interest my sister. Exactly how can screening for the islet-cell antibody help?"

"Before the test for the antibody was available, researchers were limited to examining the aftermath of the 'crash.' It was like trying to figure out what had caused a plane crash in the days before the advent of the Black Box. That specific information about an airplane's course, altitude, speed and other conditions before the crash is invaluable in reconstructing an accurate picture of what led to the crash.

"Now, by monitoring changes in the islet-cell antibody test and blood insulin levels over time, diabetes researchers can piece together an accurate picture of the events that precede the 'crash' of the beta cell. That information will eventually lead us to clues about how to prevent the crash. Islet-cell antibody testing has already revealed a very important piece of information—namely, that Type I diabetes develops over a period of several years."

"Not for me, Doc! My diabetes actually came on very suddenly. One day I was perfectly fine, doing everything I had always done. Almost overnight I was drinking everything I could get my hands on and urinating constantly—eating everything in sight but losing weight. That change only took a couple of weeks, not years."

"I know what you're saying, Mike. I was actually taught in medical school that Type I diabetes had a very rapid onset. But all those symptoms that come on so rapidly actually start at about the time of the 'crash.' The beta cells have, in fact, been in a nose dive for a long time before the symptoms occur. There are people who have gone for as long as ten years from the time they were found to have islet-cell antibodies until their diabetes developed. They felt fine until right before the diagnosis was made, but their level of insulin production had been falling with every year that passed."

"How could they be making less insulin but still be having normal blood sugars and feeling fine?"

"We think it's because the body has a relatively huge supply of beta cells, compared with the need for insulin. Researchers now are estimating that as many as 90% of the cells have to be destroyed before the blood sugar level begins to rise. In other words, once the blood sugar is truly abnormal, almost all the beta cells have already been destroyed."

"So you think my sister should get the islet-cell antibody test?"*

"Yes, Mike, I do. Using information from enough people like your sister—people who have brothers, sisters, parents or children with Type I diabetes— researchers may be able to decipher the whole process of beta cell destruction and eventually come up with a way to prevent it."

*Various research centers, including the Joslin Clinic in Boston, Massachusetts, can perform islet-cell antibody testing for relatives of persons throughout the country with Type I diabetes. You may call the Joslin Clinic, (617) 732-2546, for more information.

RESEARCH DONE NOW MAY STOP DIABETES IN THE FUTURE.

Now the darkness only stays at nighttime.
In the morning it will fade away.
Daylight is good at arriving at the right time.

George Harrison

CHAPTER 13

Is there a History of Death in Your Family? Complications

It was Sunday evening. With the weekend drawing to a close, the young man decided to walk along the beach and watch the sunset. The sky was clear except for a few lazy clouds hanging motionless near the horizon. The bright yellow glare of the afternoon sun was softening to a gold and pink glow.

As he walked along the sand, he noticed a familiar form sitting on some rocks near the water's edge. The young man's doctor was gazing silently across the bay at the setting sun.

"Hi, Doc."

"Hi, Mike."

"What are you up to?" the young man asked.

"Oh, just sitting here thinking."

"About what?"

"Life, actually. Sometimes I come down here to think about life. It helps put things in perspective."

"Perspective?"

"Well, I see a lot of people in the course of a day—often at times when things aren't going too well. They're sick and they're worried or scared. Or someone they care about is sick. And sometimes they share their deepest thoughts and concerns with me. I get to see a side of life that most people don't."

"I imagine that's pretty hard to take sometimes."

"Yes it is. But, on the other hand, it gives me a unique viewpoint on life."

"What have you learned from that?"

"Quite a bit, I think. Especially about how people respond when life throws them a curve. Different people do respond in different ways."

"I can tell you how I responded to being told I had diabetes. I got depressed. Actually I was real scared at first. And then I got angry. Since then I've been mostly frustrated. It's been a lot better since I've learned to take care of myself, but it still gets me down. Especially when I think about the long-term picture."

"I understand," the doctor replied. "A lot of my patients have told me about similar feelings. But what's really amazing to me—what really makes me think about my own outlook on life—is how some of my patients turn that situation around to their own advantage."

"Give me a break, Doc. You can't tell me there's anything good about having diabetes. It's a royal pain in the rump."

"Yeah, there's no doubt diabetes is a hard hand to play. But some people who have been dealt that particular hand seem to play it awfully well. They eat better and get more exercise than they did before. They live each day to the fullest. It's as if, for some people, the diabetes is a reminder to push ahead and live well. And then there are others who seem to see the diabetes as something that holds them back."

"It's a good point, Doc. Nobody's life is perfect. You have to play the hand you're dealt. But every time I pick up a book about diabetes I'm reminded of those long-term complications. I feel like the clock is running, and it's just a matter of time until the complications start. I often ask myself, 'When will my eyes start to bother me? How long will my kidneys last?' Some of the numbers are truly frightening."

"Well, this is a subject I talk with my patients about quite often. It's another place where perspective is really important. To put your concern about complications in perspective, we need to talk about two things: One is the way diabetes care has changed in the last few years and the other is the history of death in your family."

"How has diabetes care changed?"

"Well, if you go back as far as 1921, before insulin was available, the diagnosis of diabetes meant death in six months to two years. But insulin rewrote the book, and people survived—survived long enough to develop the complications we're so familiar with.

"Those frightening numbers you talked about earlier—the ones quoted as the likelihood you'll develop a certain complication in a given number of years and so forth—were developed between the 1920's and the 1980's, a period when the standard of diabetes management was very different from what it is today.

"Now, with patients actively involved in their own care and so many technical advances at our disposal, we can achieve much better blood sugar control than was possible at the time those statistics were compiled. Together with control of cholesterol and blood pressure, better blood sugar control can work to prevent or at the very least delay the tissue damage that leads to the long-term complications of diabetes. I think we're going to rewrite the book again in the 1990's."

"That makes a lot of sense to me, Doc. But what do you mean, 'the history of death in my family?' Everyone has a history of death in their family."

"Exactly!" the doctor answered. "Everyone is going to die. All of your ancestors have done it, and you're going to do it too. And the same would be true even if you didn't have diabetes. Everyone will die of something. And all of us—whether we have diabetes or not—have some tendency to develop health problems as we get older. How much of a tendency—or 'risk'—we have varies.

"One of the things that affects how susceptible we are to health problems as we age is how good a job we did of picking our parents—in other words, our genetic tendencies. If we picked parents who made the mistake of dying at a young age of heart disease, our risk is greater than if we'd been smart enough to pick parents who lived to a ripe old age. Now, of course, I'm kidding you a bit, since we don't actually get the chance to pick our parents.

"The point is this: As we age we all have some degree of increased risk for health problems we don't have any control over. Diabetes adds to that risk. But it doesn't make health problems a certainty.

"On the other hand, there ARE things that influence risk that we DO have control over: eating well, staying physically active, avoiding smoking and substance abuse, keeping weight down, and keeping blood pressure and blood sugar under control. These are things we can do to minimize whatever risk we have inherited from our parents or acquired through developing diabetes."

"I think you're right," replied the young man. "I guess whether we have diabetes or not, we only have so much tread on our tires. And it's a matter of trying to get the most mileage possible out of the tread we've got."

"Now you're telling stories too," the doctor observed. "Think you've spent too much time with us?"

"Not really. Sometimes the stories help me see things more clearly. They get the point across."

"It's too late now to go back and pick different parents to improve your chances for a healthy old age. And you can't get rid of your diabetes just yet—although you may see that happen in your lifetime. So, as the old philosopher says, 'A wise man accepts what he can't change.'

"But the things you CAN change—the things you DO have control over—how healthfully you eat, how much you exercise, how well you control your blood sugar, blood pressure and cholesterol, whether or not you smoke, whether or not you wear your seat belt when you get in your car, and so on—are well worth your effort. Those are things that help you get the most mileage out of the tread you've got. They can make a difference. And that's just as true for people who don't have diabetes as it is for those who do.

"Remember your family not only has a history of death, it also has a history of LIFE!

"Go out and live it well."

THERE IS HOPE.

YOU HAVE CONTROL!

INDEX

Additional copies of this book can be obtained by
sending $7.95 plus $2 for shipping and handling to:

Diabetes 101
c/o Diabetes Center, Inc.
P.O. Box 739
Wayzata, Minnesota 55391

Order forms can be obtained and orders
for additional books can be placed by calling
1-612-541-0239.

HEALTH PROFESSIONALS:
Contact us for special educational discounts.

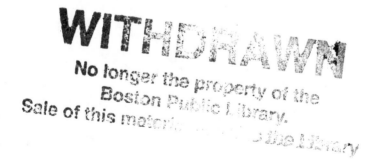

If you found this book helpful and would like more information on this and other related subjects, you may be interested in one or more of the following titles from our *Wellness and Nutrition Library.*

BOOKS
Expresslane Diet: (176 pages)
Retirement: New Beginnings, New Challenges, New Successes (140 pages)
Whole Parent/Whole Child: Raising a Chronically Ill Child (175 pages)
Diabetes: A Guide to Living Well (365 pages)
D. A. S. H. Diabetes . . . Actively Staying Healthy (220 pages)
Adult Braces in a Gourmet World (148 pages)
I Can Cope: Staying Healthy with Cancer (202 pages)
Managing Type II Diabetes (148 pages)
Managing the School Age Child with a Chronic Health Condition (350 pages)
Pass the Pepper Please (66 pages)
The Guiltless Gourmet (170 pages)
The Joy of Snacks (270 pages)
Fast Food Facts (56 pages)
Convenience Food Facts (188 pages)
Learning to Live Well With Diabetes (392 pages)
The Physician Within (170 pages)
Exchanges for All Occasions (250 pages)
Opening the Door to Good Nutrition (186 pages)

BOOKLETS & PAMPHLETS
Eating with Food Choices (40 pages)
A Guide to Healthy Eating (60 pages)
Diabetes & Alcohol (4 pages)
Diabetes & Exercise (20 pages)
Emotional Adjustment to Diabetes (16 pages)
A Step In Time: Diabetes Foot Care (18 pages)
Diabetes Record Book (68 pages)
Diabetes & Brief Illness (8 pages)
Diabetes & Impotence: A Concern for Couples (6 pages)
Adding Fiber to Your Diet (10 pages)
Gestational Diabetes: Guidelines for a Safe Pregnancy (24 pages)
Recognizing and Treating Insulin Reactions (4 pages)
Hypoglycemia (functional) (4 pages)

PROFESSIONAL SERIES
Manual of Clinical Nutrition (540 pages)
Simplified Learning Series: 17-booklet preview packet
Diabetes Youth Curriculum: For working with young patients, ages 6 to 16.

The Wellness and Nutrition Library is published by Diabetes Center, Inc., in Minneapolis, MN, publishers of quality educational materials dealing with health, wellness, nutrition, diabetes, and other chronic illnesses. All our books and materials are available nationwide and in Canada through leading bookstores. If you can't find our books at your favorite bookstore, contact us directly for a free catalog.

DCI Publishing, Inc.
P.O. Box 739
Wayzata, MN 55391

DIABETES 101:
Candy Apples, Log Cabins & You

In this simple guide for people with insulin dependent diabetes the authors, experts in diabetes care and education, use visual images of everyday items, such as candy apples and log cabins, to provide the basic information needed by people using insulin. Stripped of the medical/technical jargon common to so many diabetes books, this easy to read book will be welcomed by the newly diagnosed and their families, as well as the skilled health professional.

"Many of the books about diabetes are written in a clinical style at a level of understanding that may create more confusion than knowledge or inspiration. Finally, here is a book that is fun to read and is full of practical, relevant information of how a person with diabetes can meet the challenge of daily living. *Diabetes 101* should be read by everyone who has diabetes or who is a family member of someone with diabetes and by all health care providers that work in the field of diabetes. You will not only learn from this book, but you will be touched in a positive way by the authors' understanding, sensitivity and ability to teach and entertain you. I highly recommend this unique book."
R. Keith Campbell, R.Ph., F.A.P.P., C.D.E., *Associate Dean & Professor of Pharmacy Practice*, Washington State University

"As a 24 year old, recently diagnosed with diabetes, this book gave me a clear understanding of diabetes. The authors' insights and explanations gave me a realistic picture of potential problems and offered understandable solutions to acquiring better blood sugar control. This is an excellent book and its down-to-earth approach provided me with a "soup-to-nuts" survival guide."
Mark Harnois, *Newly diagnosed with diabetes*, Scottsdale, AZ

"The unique, narrative style of *Diabetes 101* makes the practical and accurate information it contains easy to both understand and remember."
George Eisenbarth, M.D., Ph.D., *Chief, Section of Immunology*
Joslin Diabetes Center, Boston, MA
Associate Professor, Dept. of Medicine, Harvard Medical School

"This manual will be very useful to any person who has diabetes mellitus. Its clear, conversational style make it easy to understand as it provides practical applications for living daily with diabetes."
Warner Burch, M.D., *Associate Professor of Medicine*
Duke University Medical Center

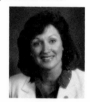 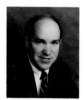

Betty Brackenridge, M.S., R.D., C.D.E., and **Richard O. Dolinar, M.D.,** practice together in Phoenix, Arizona, integrating diabetes medical care with diabetes self-care education in Dr. Dolinar's endocrinology practice. He is Director of Diabetes Research for the Human Diabetes Center of Excellence in Phoenix. Ms. Brackenridge is President of the American Association of Diabetes Educators.

ISBN 0-937721-63-8   DCI Publishing $7.9
HEALT